EMQs for MRCOG
Part 2 in Gynaecology

Authors

Prabha Sinha
FRCOG, MRCPI, Dip Med Ed, Dip Mgmt
Consultant Obstetrician and Gynaecologist
East Sussex Hospitals NHS Trust

Mamta Mishra
MS, MRCOG

Consultant Obstetrician and Gynaecologist
Fortis Hospital New Delhi, India

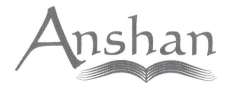

EMQs FOR MRCOG PART 2 IN GYNAECOLOGY

Published by:
Anshan Ltd
6 Newlands Road
Tunbridge Wells
Kent. TN1 1YS

Tel: +44 (0) 1892 557767
Fax: +44 (0) 1892 530358

e-mail: info@anshan.co.uk
website: www.anshan.co.uk

ISBN: 9781848290778

British Library Cataloguing in Publication Data

A catalogue record for this book is available from the British Library.

Every effort has been made to trace all copyright holders, but if any have been inadvertently overlooked the publishers will be pleased to make the necessary arrangements at the first opportunity.

Copy Editor: Catherine Lain
Cover Design: Emma Randall
Cover Image: Shutterstock
Typeset by: Kerrypress Typesetters, Luton, Bedfordshire
Printed and bound by:

Contents

Preface

The Royal College of Obstetricians and Gynaecologists (RCOG) introduced Extended Matching Questions (EMQs) some time ago, partially replacing the old-style MCQs and short essays. As EMQs provide greater consistency and fairness, are more transparent and test the depth of knowledge of the candidates in the exam, more emphasis has been put on them.

Generally EMQs are very similar to multiple choice questions. However, the main difference is that EMQs test the depth of applied knowledge, making the exams more authentic, transparent and valid. The probability of getting the correct answer by chance is very low and therefore candidates must have an adequate knowledge prior to attempting the questions.

From March 2011 the format of the Part 2 MRCOG written examination has changed and the number of EMQs has increased from 40 to 90. EMQs now make up 40% of overall marks whereas before they only accounted for 15%. There are three papers in the written examination. The number of questions and the time allotted to answer them have been changed accordingly.

The distribution of the marks is as follows (RCOG website):

	Proportion of Overall Marks
Paper 1 (4 SAQs) – 105 minutes	30%
Paper 2 (120 MCQs, 45 EMQs) – 135 minutes	30%
Paper 3 (120 MCQs, 45 EMQs) – 135 minutes	40%

As this book contains evidence-based answers, candidates will find them easy to follow. The book features 151 questions covering most of the subject of gynaecological practice and is primarily based on guidelines published by the RCOG, the National Institute for Health and Clinical Excellence (NICE) and the most up-to-date research and consensus.

All the questions are based on real clinical scenarios commonly encountered in day-to-day clinical practice such as that from outpatient clinics, acute admissions from accident and emergency and gynaecology wards.

It is essential to practice EMQs before taking the exam. However, basic detailed knowledge is necessary and studying textbooks is required to gain knowledge in preparation for the exam. Books such as those containing short essays, MCQs and EMQs are not a replacement for textbooks. This book will coach students to answer EMQs effectively once they have acquired a basic knowledge. Revision of the guidelines should ensue.

Full details about the exam itself are available on the RCOG website. This book follows the established format; just choose the most appropriate answer for each question. It is important to read the statements carefully to identify the theme and then select the most relevant and appropriate answer.

For the revision of the Part 2 MRCOG exam this book is essential.

Syllabus

The syllabus is freely available on the RCOG website. It is comprised of 19 modules and includes basic clinical and surgical skills, audit, research, clinical risk (clinical governance), teaching and appraisal.

In gynaecology the main modules include detailed knowledge regarding common gynaecological diseases, infertility/subfertility, contraception and sexual health, pelvic floor (including urological problems), oncology and perioperative and post-operative care.

These modules are based on standard textbooks and guidelines, teaching material provided by the RCOG e.g. TOG, StratOG, DIALOG.

Examination preparation not only includes detailed subject knowledge but also that of recent evidence related to the subject, published in the greentop guidelines by RCOG, NICE and other relevant places (CEMACH, National Screening).

Journals such as BJOG and TOG are also relevant as they too discuss recent development.

Abbreviations

A&E	Accident and Emergency
AFP	Alfa feto protein
ANOVA	Analysis of variance
BMI	Body mass index
BP	Blood pressure
BSO	Bilateral salpingo-oophorectomy
CEU	Clinical effectiveness unit
CS	Caesarean section
CT	Computed tomographic scan
CTG	Cardiotocographic
CRL	Crown-rump length
D&C	Dilatation and curettage
DUB	Dysfunctional uterine bleeding
EP	Ectopic pregnancy
EPAU	Early pregnancy assessment unit
ERCP	Endoscopic retrograde cholangiopancreatography
FIGO	International Federation of Gynaecology and Obstetrics
FSH	Follicle stimulating hormone
GCT	Granulosa cell tumour
GnRH	Gonadotropin-releasing hormone
GP	General Practitioner
GTD	Gestational trophoblastic disease
GTN	Gestational trophoblastic neoplasia
hCG	Human chorionic gonadotropin
HIV	Human immunodeficiency virus
HMB	Heavy menstrual bleeding
hMG	Human menopausal gonadotropin
HRT	Hormone replacement therapy
HyCoSy	Hystero-salpingo contrast sonography
ICSI	Intra-cytoplasmic sperm injection
IEP	Interstitial ectopic pregnancies
IOTA	International Ovarian Tumor Analysis

IUD	Intrauterine device
IUGR	Intrauterine growth restriction
IVF	In vitro fertilization
LDL	Low density lipoprotein
LH	Luteinising hormone
LLETZ	Large loop excision of transformation zone
LMP	Last missed period
LNG-IUS	Levonorgestrel-releasing intrauterine system
LSCS	Lower section caesarean section
MRI	Magnetic resonance imaging
MSD	Mean gestational sac diameter
NSAIDs	Nonsteroidal anti-inflammatory drugs
NPV	Negative predictive value
OHSS	Ovarian hyperstimulation syndrome
PCOS	Polycystic ovary syndrome
PD	Paget's disease
PGD	Pre-implantation genetic diagnosis
PID	Pelvic inflammatory disease
PPV	Positive predictive value
PUL	Pregnancy of unknown location
RMI	Risk of malignancy index
SHO	Senior House Officer
SROM	Spontaneous rupture of membrane
SSRI	Selective serotonin reuptake inhibitor
TAH	Total abdominal hysterectomy
TESE	Testicular sperm extraction
TOA	Tubo-ovarian abscess
TORCH	Toxoplasma, rubella, cytomegalovirus and herpes virus
TRUS	Transrectal ultrasound
TVS	Transvaginal scan
USG	Ultrasound
VIN	Vulval intraepithelial neoplasia
VTE	Venous thromboembolism

About the authors

Prabha Sinha is a Consultant Obstetrician and Gynaecologist at the Conquest Hospital in St Leonards-on-Sea, East Sussex, UK. She is also Honorary Consultant in Fetal Medicine at Guy's and St. Thomas' Hospitals in London. She has Fellowship of the Royal College of Obstetricians and Gynaecologists (FRCOG) and Membership of the Royal College of Physicians of Ireland (MRCPI). She is involved with undergraduate students from Brighton and GKT Medical School, as well as postgraduate education and assessment. She is currently an examiner for the Membership of the Royal College of Obstetricians and Gynaecologists (MRCOG), as well as the GMC exam for overseas doctors. She has also been a teacher on MRCOG courses locally, nationally, at the RCOG and internationally.

She has published many articles in peer reviewed journals and made a huge number of presentations and lectures in various national and international conferences.

She has written EMQ books for MRCOG Part 1, 2, DRCOG and OSCE for Colposcopy.

This is her ninth authored book.

Dr Mamta Mishra is a senior consultant at Fortis Hospital at New Delhi in India. She has vast experience in obstetrics and gynaecology and a great interest in teaching and training. She has published many articles and made a number of presentations at various national and international conferences. She is actively involved in organising conferences and courses for MRCOG Part 1 and 2 twice a year in New Delhi. She has co-written books on consent issues and EMQs based on guidelines in obstetrics. This is her third book.

EMQs on Early Pregnancy Complications

Options for questions 1 – 3

A	Oral glucose tolerance test	H	Thyroid function tests
B	Hyperprolactinemia	I	Reassurance
C	Blood sugar	J	TORCH screening
D	Peripheral blood karyotyping of parents before cytogenetic analysis of product of conception	K	Screening for antiphospholipid antibody (lupus anticoagulant, anticardiolipin antibody etc.)
E	Routine screening for thyroid antibodies	L	Cytogenetic analysis of product of conception
F	Pelvic USG	M	Thrombophilia screen
G	Peripheral blood karyotyping	N	Endometrial biopsy

Instruction: For each option posed above, choose the single most appropriate investigation from the A-N list. The given option may be used once, more than once or not at all.

Question 1	A 28 year P0+3 has been referred to the clinic by her GP. She has a history of recurrent miscarriage at 6, 8 and 10 weeks. Her USG scan is normal.
Question 2	A 36 year old woman has been admitted via A&E with bleeding per vaginum and 8 weeks of amenorrhea. This is her fourth pregnancy. She had been investigated for recurrent miscarriage before and no cause had been ascertained. She is now going for an ERPC for an incomplete miscarriage.
Question 3	A 28 year old woman is very anxious as she has had 3 miscarriages in the past. You noticed that she miscarried at 15, 6 and 8 weeks. Her scan is normal and screening for antiphospholipid antibody syndrome is negative.

Answers and explanations

Answer 1 (K) Screening for antiphospholipid antibody
(lupus anticoagulant, anticardiolipin antibody etc.)

Antiphospholipid antibodies are present in 15% of women with recurrent miscarriages. Lupus anticoagulant, anti-B2 glycoprotein-1 antibodies and anticardiolipin antibodies are collectively called antiphospholipid antibodies.

It is a hypercoaguable state due to an alteration in the clotting mechanism, which can affect any organ. In pregnancy it is associated with recurrent miscarriage, pre-eclampsia, IUGR, preterm delivery and intrauterine death.

Antiphospholipid syndrome is characterized by the presence of antiphospholipid antibodies in a woman who has had the adverse pregnancy outcomes below:

- three or more consecutive miscarriages before 10 weeks
- one or more morphologically normal foetal losses after the 10th week
- one or more preterm births before 34 weeks of gestation due to placental disease.

It is essential to have two positive tests at least 12 weeks apart for lupus anticoagulant or anticardiolipin antibodies of immunoglobulin G and/ or immunoglobulin M. The titre should be present in a medium or high range over 40 g/l or ml/l or above the 99th percentile.

Answer 2 (L) Cytogenetic analysis of product of conception

Recent evidence suggests that karyotyping of couples is recommended if a chromosomal abnormality is detected in the product of conception. Hence, in women with recurrent miscarriage, cytogenetic analysis on the product of conception should be done to look for unbalanced structural chromosomal abnormalities.

Answer 3 (M) Thrombophilia screen

Inherited thrombophilias such as Factor V Leiden, Factor II (prothrombin) gene mutation and protein S deficiency have been found to be associated with second trimester miscarriage. Therefore, a woman with one previous second trimester miscarriage should be screened for these defects.

Options for questions 4 – 7

A	Genetic counselling	G	Progesterone
B	Aspirin alone	H	Bromocriptine
C	Heparin alone	I	Immunotherapy
D	Aspirin and steroids	J	Aspirin and heparin
E	History indicated cervical cerclage	K	Peri-implantation genetic diagnosis
F	USG indicated cervical cerclage	L	Transvaginal sonographic surveillance of cervical length

Instruction: For each question posed below, choose the single most appropriate management from the A-L list above. The given option may be used once, more than once or not at all.

Question 4	A 26 year old P1+1 is seen in the clinic. She is currently 12 weeks pregnant. She had a premature delivery two years ago at 26 weeks. After that her second pregnancy ended in a miscarriage at 16 weeks.
Question 5	A 26 year old woman G5 P0+4 is seen in the outpatient clinic. She is 6 weeks pregnant. Previous obstetric history includes one termination of pregnancy and three recurrent miscarriages at 6, 8 and 8 weeks gestation. She was investigated and found to have lupus anticoagulant titre of 80 g/l on 2 occasions.
Question 6	A 28 year old woman has had three miscarriages at 15, 6 and 8 weeks. Her scan is normal and screening for antiphospholipid syndrome is negative. She is found to be positive for the Factor V gene variant.
Question 7	A 39 year old woman has miscarried for the third time and has had an ERPC. It was an IVF conception. Cytogenetic analysis has suggested translocation. Parental karyotyping confirmed them to be a carrier for translocation.

Answer (4) L Transvaginal sonographic surveillance of cervical length

In women with a history of two or fewer previous preterm births or second trimester losses, 'history indicated' cerclage is not offered. A history such as painless dilatation or the onset of contractions after the rupture of membranes should not be used as reasons to offer cerclage. Instead, history-indicated cerclage is offered to a woman who has three or more previous preterm births and/or second trimester losses. Transvaginal sonographic surveillance of cervical length should be offered to women who have a history of preterm birth and/or mid-trimester loss. If the length of the cervix is less than 25 mm before 24 weeks, then USG-guided cervical cerclage should be offered.

Answer 5 (J) Aspirin and heparin

Evidence suggests that aspirin along with heparin is the only treatment that significantly improves the chance of live birth rates in women who are diagnosed to have antiphospholipid syndrome. It reduces the miscarriage rate by 50–60%.

Heparin does not cross the placental barrier so there is no risk to the foetus. Maternal side effects of heparin include hypersensitivity, osteopenia and thrombocytopenia. The adverse effects are minimal if low molecular weight heparin is used.

Answer 6 (C) Heparin alone

Evidence does not very strongly recommend giving heparin to women who have recurrent first trimester miscarriages and are found to be positive for inherited thrombophilia such as protein S deficiency, prothrombin gene variant, or Factor V Leiden deficiency. But it has been suggested that treatment with heparin therapy may improve the live birth rate in women who have had second trimester miscarriage and have inherited the thrombophilia defect.

Answer 7 (K) Pre-implantation genetic diagnosis (PGD)

Recurrent miscarriage is known to be associated with parental chromosomal abnormalities, particularly balanced reciprocal and Robertsonian translocations. PGD improves the pregnancy outcome of translocation carriers with a history of repeated pregnancy loss.
This conception was due to IVF. As the woman has got chromosomal rearrangements, she should be offered PGD.

Patients should be counselled that IVF with PGD/PGS may result in a lower pregnancy rate due to a reduction in the number of chromosomally normal embryos available for embryo transfer (see RCOG, *Green-top Guideline* no. 17).

Options for questions 8 – 10

A	Incomplete miscarriage	F	Spontaneous miscarriage
B	Complete miscarriage	G	Threatened miscarriage
C	Missed miscarriage	H	Miscarriage with infection
D	Pregnancy of uncertain viability	I	Pregnancy of unknown location
E	Inevitable miscarriage	J	Recurrent miscarriage

Instruction: For each question posed below, choose the single most appropriate diagnosis from the A-J list above. The given option may be used once, more than once or not at all.

Question 8	A 35 year old G2 has attended the EPAU as her urine pregnancy test is positive. She is not sure of her dates. She is very anxious as she has previously had a miscarriage at 7 weeks. On the TVS there are no signs of either intrauterine or extrauterine or retained product of conception. She has been bleeding for the last 3 days. Her βhCG, which was repeated twice in 48 hours, has gone up from 405 to 662.
Question 9	A 30 year old G4 P1+3 has attended the EPAU as she has had some spotting and a dull ache in her lower abdomen. She thinks she is 7 weeks pregnant. The TVS scan showed an intrauterine sac of 16 mm x 14 mm x 12 mm with no obvious yolk sac or foetus. Her blood sample has been taken for serum βhCG and progesterone.
Question 10	A 26 year old G2 P0+1 has attended the EPAU as she has had some spotting. The TVS scan showed an intrauterine sac of 20 mm x 18 mm x 22 mm with a foetus with a crown-lump length of 6 mm. She has had an ectopic pregnancy previously and a left salpingectomy was performed.

Answers and explanations

Answer 8 (I) Pregnancy of unknown location

A pregnancy of unknown location (PUL) is a term used when a woman has a positive pregnancy test but no intra or extra-uterine pregnancy is visualised on transvaginal sonography. Outcomes of PULs include intrauterine pregnancy, miscarriages and ectopic pregnancy.

Expectant management has been shown to be safe for the majority of women with a PUL. Further management includes serum progesterone and human chorionic gonadotropin level monitoring which helps in making a diagnosis.

Answer 9 (D) Pregnancy of uncertain viability

Intrauterine pregnancy of uncertain viability (PUV) is defined as the transvaginal sonographic (TVS) visualization of a small intrauterine gestational sac without the demonstration of cardiac activity in the embryo.

The finding can indicate a normal early pregnancy of approximately 4–6 weeks gestational age or a failed or failing pregnancy with arrested or reduced growth, which is destined to miscarry. The criteria that is used to diagnose early pregnancy failure varies. In the United Kingdom, guidelines state that the diagnosis of pregnancy failure may be made when the mean gestational sac diameter (MSD) exceeds 25 mm with no visible embryonic pole, or the embryonic crown-rump length (CRL) is greater than 7 mm with no visible heart pulsation. Whichever cut-off values are used, the diagnosis of miscarriage is subsequently made if an embryonic heartbeat is not visible on the TVS after an interval of at least 7 days. This interval assessment aims to prevent the misdiagnosis of a potentially viable pregnancy as a miscarriage and thus minimise the chance of an inadvertent termination of pregnancy.

Answer 10 (D) Pregnancy of uncertain viability

See explanation as above.

Options for questions 11 – 13

A	Mefipristone and misoprostol	G	Reassurance
B	Surgical management with antibiotic cover	H	Repeat scan after one week
C	Surgical management	I	Misoprostol alone
D	Expectant management	J	Diagnostic laparoscopy
E	Methotrexate	K	Antibiotics
F	Repeat scan after 2 weeks	L	Repeat scan after 3 weeks

Instruction: For each question posed below, choose the single most appropriate answer from the A-L list above. The given option may be used once, more than once or not at all.

Question 11	A 26 year old primigravida had a scan done which suggested a missed miscarriage at 8 weeks. She opted for medical management. Four weeks later she attended with continuing bleeding and was unwell. On examination her temperature was 38, pulse 110/min and BP was 110/60 mmHG. A scan done suggests a retained product measuring 40 mm x 35 mm x 26 mm.
Question 12	A 15 year old primigravida has attended the EPAU as she has had some spotting. She is not sure of her LMP. A TV scan showed an intrauterine sac of 20 mm x 18 mm x 23 mm in diameter with no obvious yolk sac or foetus. Her βhCG is 1000 IU/L.
Question 13	A 22 year old G6 P4+1 has come to A&E complaining of excessive bleeding per vaginum. Her periods were irregular. On examination her pulse is 110/min, BP is 94/60 mmHg. A vaginal examination shows bleeding ++. Further examination was stopped as it was very painful. A pregnancy test is positive.

Answers and explanations

Answer 11 (B) Surgical management with antibiotic cover

Women are increasingly offered a choice of treatment for the management of miscarriage. Expectant and medical management should be offered only in units where patients have access to 24 hour telephone advice and immediate admission can be arranged. Surgical evacuation remains the treatment of choice if endometrial thickness is >50 mm and bleeding is excessive, vital signs are unstable or infected tissue is present in the uterine cavity (in which case surgery must be done under antibiotic cover).

Rare surgical risks are:

- uterine perforation (1%)
- cervical tears
- intra-abdominal trauma (0.1%)
- intrauterine adhesions
- haemorrhage
- infection
- anaesthetic complications.

Answer 12 (H) Repeat scan after one week

The diagnosis in this case is intrauterine pregnancy of uncertain viability (PUV). The finding can indicate a normal early pregnancy of approximately 4–6 weeks gestational age or a failed or failing pregnancy. The scan should be repeated in a week's time. This interval assessment aims to prevent the misdiagnosis of a potentially viable pregnancy as a miscarriage and thus minimise the chance of an inadvertent termination of the pregnancy.

Answer 13 (C) Surgical management

In this case, bleeding is excessive and the woman is haemodynamically unstable, therefore the surgical management is acceptable.
(Ref. RCOP, *Green-top Guideline* no. 25.)

Options for questions 14 – 16

A	18 months from normalisation of the βhCG level	G	18 months from the date of uterine evacuation
B	βhCG level to be checked immediately	H	Weekly βhCG till it reaches below 2 IU
C	6 months from normalisation of the βhCG level	I	6 months from the date of uterine evacuation
D	12 months from normalisation of the βhCG level	J	βhCG level 3–4 weeks after the end of pregnancy
E	12 months from the date of uterine evacuation	K	βhCG level 6–8 weeks after the end of pregnancy
F	Follow-up not required	L	Bi-weekly βhCG level

Instruction: For each question posed below, choose the single most appropriate time to follow them up from the A-L list above. The given option may be used once, more than once or not at all.

Question 14	An 18 year old woman primigravida has had a suction evacuation done for molar pregnancy. She is being followed up and her serum βhCG has reverted to normal within 56 days of the uterine evacuation.
Question 15	A 35 year old woman was diagnosed to have molar pregnancy in the scan done in the EPAU. She had a suction evacuation and was registered for follow-up. Her serum βhCG has not reverted to normal within 56 days of the uterine evacuation of molar pregnancy.
Question 16	A 39 year old G2 was admitted to the labour ward at 36 weeks into her pregnancy with a history of SROM. She was contracting 3 in 10 and delivered 6 hours after admission. She wants to have a 6 hour discharge. It has just been noticed that her previous pregnancy 3 years ago was a molar pregnancy

Answers and explanations

Answer 14 (I) 6 months from the date of uterine evacuation

Follow-up is mandatory in all women with gestational trophoblastic disease to rule out the possibility of persistent disease, to diagnose early malignant uterine invasion or malignant metastatic disease. Following uterine evacuation, 18–29% of patients with a complete hydatidiform mole and 1–11% of patients with a partial hydatidiform mole develop a persistent trophoblastic tumour.

βhCG levels are checked every 2 weeks to see if the level is falling or not. If the βhCG falls to normal within 8 weeks of evacuation, the monitoring can be stopped at 6 months post evacuation.

If the βhCG falls more slowly, monitoring can stop at 6 months following the first normal value after normalisation. Monitoring is done by urine βhCG monthly after normalisation of the serum βhCG.

It is deemed to be persistent when βhCG is still elevated after 16 weeks of evacuation. Sharp regression is when levels immediately fall after evacuation. Slow regression is seen as when serum levels regress slowly to normal within 8 to 9 weeks from the uterine evacuation.

FIGO indications for chemotherapy treatment are:

1. βhCG plateau of 4 values +/- 10% over a 3 week period
2. βhCG increase of >10% of three values over a 2 week period
3. Persistence of βhCG for more than 6 months after molar.

Answer 15 (C) 6 months from normalisation of the βhCG level

The duration of monitoring varies depending on when the levels reach normal. If the level gets to normal within 56 days following the evacuation then the monitoring continues for a total of 6 months from the day of the evacuation. In those patients where the βhCG level takes more than 56 days, the monitoring goes on for 6 months from the date of the first normal sample. In both situations it is advised that a further pregnancy is deferred until the end of the follow-up period as the pregnancy may mask evidence of the relapse of the illness. This can happen in a very small number of women.

The risk of developing a future second molar pregnancy is approximately 1 in 80. The surge of hormones in a later pregnancy can cause a relapse of the old molar pregnancy and start any cells still present to grow again and potentially cause problems. Whilst this problem is very rare, urine should be tested 6 weeks after delivery. Four weeks later, urine and blood tests should be repeated.

Answer 16 (K) βhCG level 6–8 weeks after the end of the pregnancy

Patients with molar disease are at an increased risk of developing a molar pregnancy in subsequent conceptions. After one molar pregnancy, the risk of having molar disease in a future conception is about 1%. The risk of developing molar disease in a subsequent conception is 15–20% in patients with two molar pregnancies.

However, patients with repeat mole can achieve normal full-term pregnancies. Because of the increased risk of later molar disease, βhCG should be measured 6 weeks after the completion of any future pregnancy to exclude choriocarcinoma.

Options for questions 17 – 18

A	Intrauterine contraceptive device	F	Progesterone-only emergency pill
B	Check serum hCG and continue with oral contraception	G	May continue with oral contraception
C	Hormone replacement therapy	H	Combined oral contraception
D	Stop oral contraception	I	Barrier contraception
E	Contraception not required	J	LNG-IUS

Instruction: For each question posed below, choose the single most appropriate safe contraception from the A-J list above. The given option may be used once, more than once or not at all.

Question 17	A 22 year old woman has had an ERPC done for suspected missed miscarriage. The surgeon noticed a grape-like structure during surgery. Histology confirmed it to be a molar pregnancy. She is seen in the clinic and is shocked to hear the diagnosis. She is seeking contraceptive advice.
Question 18	A 36 year old woman has started oral contraception after evacuation for an incomplete miscarriage. Histological assessment of the product of conception confirmed it to be gestational trophoblastic disease (GTD). What contraceptive would be suitable for her?

Answers and explanations

Answer 17 (I) Barrier contraception

Patients with a molar pregnancy must be encouraged to use reliable contraception during the entire interval of βhCG monitoring. An intrauterine device should be avoided before gonadotropin remission because of the risk of uterine perforation with invasive tumour. Oral contraceptives increase the frequency of post-molar tumours two-to-three fold if used prior to gonadotropin remission.

Answer 18 (G) May continue with oral contraception

Women with GTD should be advised to use barrier methods of contraception until βhCG levels revert to normal.

The combined oral contraceptive pill may be used. If this has been started before the diagnosis of GTD was made, the woman can continue to remain on oral contraception. However, she should be advised that there is a potential (but low increased) risk of developing gestational trophoblastic neoplasia (GTN). There is no evidence as to whether single-agent progestogens have any effect on GTN.
(Ref. RCOG, *Green-top Guideline* no. 38.)

Options for questions 19 – 21

A	Expectant management	F	Reassurance
B	Medical management	G	Laparotomy
C	Laparoscopic salpingostomy	H	Serial βhCG
D	Laparoscopic salpingectomy	I	Discharge
E	KCl	J	Serum progesterone

Instruction: For each question posed below, choose the single most appropriate answer from the A-J list above. The given option may be used once, more than once or not at all.

Question 19	A 30 year old woman came to the early pregnancy unit with slight bleeding. Her LMP was 5 weeks ago and a pregnancy test was positive. Her βhCG was 446. A transvaginal scan was normal with mild tenderness in the left adenaxe during examination. She opted for expectant management. Her repeat βhCG in 48 hours was 250. She has presented the next day with severe pain in her abdomen and feeling very unwell.
Question 20	A 26 year old woman's urine pregnancy test was positive at 6 weeks. She presented at EPAU with pain in the right adenaxe. Her βhCG was 660. A USG scan showed a right adenaxe mass of 2 cm x 3 cm in size. Her repeat βhCG in 48 hours is 333.
Question 21	A 25 year old nulliparous woman is admitted with lower abdominal pain of 2 days' duration. Her βhCG is 3621 and serum progesterone is 26. A transvaginal scan suggests a mass of 3 cm x 4 cm in the left adenaxe, with a gestational sac and cardiac activity also visualised.

Answers and explanations

Answer 19 (G) Laparotomy

In a haemodynamically unstable patient, emergency laparotomy is the most appropriate management. The indications for surgical treatment are women who are not suitable or have failed methotrexate treatment, those with heterotopic pregnancy, or those who are haemodynamically unstable. Surgical treatment includes salpingostomy or salpingectomy.

Salpingostomy preserves the tube but there is small risk of persistent trophoblast and a repeat ipsilateral tubal ectopic pregnancy.

Salpingectomy avoids these risks but leaves only one tube for reproductive capacity. Clinicians prefer a salpingectomy over a salpingostomy in the presence of a healthy contra lateral tube. This preference is based on the small risk of tubal bleeding in the immediate post-operative period. The potential need for further treatment for a persistent trophoblast and the possibility of a repeat EP is in the conserved tube. Salpingectomy is the preferred option in cases where the other tube is healthy.

Laparoscopic procedures are associated with shorter operative times, less intraoperative blood loss, shorter hospital stays and lower analgesia requirements. Laparotomy is done when women present with a rupture and are in a state of hypovolaemic shock and compromise.

Answer 20 (A) Expectant management

When the βhCG level is less than 1000 IU/L, a woman is haemodynamically stable and expectant management is the treatment of choice. The incidences of ectopic pregnancy have increased due to the highly sensitive screening test (i.e. radioimmunoassay βhCG) and transvaginal sonography. Stable, minimally symptomatic and asymptomatic patients with a positive pregnancy test and negative findings on transvaginal sonography can be followed up by measuring their quantitative βhCG level. Surgery can be avoided in a significant number of patients who would once have required operative intervention. Patients who are treated with expectant management have a good long-term fertility outcome and the risk for repeat EP is low.

Answer 21 (D) Laparoscopic salpingectomy

Medical management is contraindicated as cardiac activity is visualised, so laparoscopic salpingectomy is the treatment of choice. This is the case even if the patient is haemodynamically stable and the ectopic is live and not ruptured.

Options for questions 22 – 24

A	Until hCG levels are less than 20 IU/L	F	Twice weekly βhCG measurements and weekly TVS examinations
B	βhCG on days 4 and 7	G	Laparoscopic salpingotomy
C	Laparoscopic salpingectomy	H	Methotrexate is repeated
D	Reassurance	I	Serial serum progesterone
E	Laparotomy	J	Expectant management

Instruction: For each question posed below, choose the single most appropriate answer from the A-J list above. The given option may be used once, more than once or not at all.

Question 22	A 20 year old patient has come to the early pregnancy unit with pain in her lower abdomen. Her LMP was 6 weeks ago and a pregnancy test is positive. Her βhCG is 2600. A transvaginal scan shows a right adenaxe mass of 3 cm x 2.5 cm. She has opted for medical management. She has received intramuscular methotrexate and you are arranging her follow-up.
Question 23	A 19 year old patient has come to the early pregnancy unit with slight bleeding. Her LMP was 6 weeks ago and a pregnancy test is positive. Her βhCG is 784 IU/L. A transvaginal scan is normal with slight probe tenderness in left adenaxe. She has opted for expectant management.
Question 24	A 20 year old patient has had a βhCG of 2000 and a scan has failed to detect an intrauterine pregnancy. She has opted for medical management. She has received an injection of methotrexate. Serial βhCG measurements have failed to fall by more than 15%.

Answers and explanations

Answer 22 (B) βhCG on days 4 and 7

Indications for medical management are when a woman:

- is haemodynamically stable
- has minimal symptoms
- has a βhCG less than 3000 IU/L
- is willing to have a follow-up.

7% of women might rupture, 75% experience pain and approximately 15% might require another dose of methotrexate.

Answer 23 (F) Twice weekly βhCG measurements and weekly TVS examinations

Proper selection of cases is required for expectant management. Indications of expectant management are where:

- the woman is asymptomatic
- there is no evidence or less than 100ml of fluid in the pouch of Douglas
- the βhCG level is 1000 IU/L at the initial presentation.

Follow-up involves twice weekly βhCG level measurements and weekly transvaginal examinations. The level should decrease by more than 50% of its initial level within 7 days and the size of the mass should reduce. Follow-up is continued by weekly βhCG and scan till βhCG level falls to 20 IU/L.

Answer 24 (H) Methotrexate is repeated

The dose of methotrexate is calculated by a patient's body surface area (50 mg/m²) She is then monitored by checking βhCG on days 4 and 7. If the βhCG levels do not decrease by more than 15% between these days then the injection should be repeated.

(Ref. RCOG, *Green-top Guideline* no. 21.)

EMQs on Premenstrual Syndrome

Options for questions 25 – 27

A	Cognitive behavioural therapy	F	TAH with bilateral salpingo-oopherectomy
B	GnRH analogues along with add-back therapy	G	Low dose SSRI in luteal phase
C	Progesterone tablets	H	Vitamin B6 30mg/day
D	Light therapy	I	Cyclical contraceptive pill
E	Continuous contraceptive pill	J	Danazol

Instruction: For each question posed below, choose the single most appropriate answer from the A-J list above. The given option may be used once, more than once or not at all.

Question 25	A 42 year old woman has been seen in the clinic with symptoms of premenstrual depression and bad temper. She is on the verge of being extremely violent and has not been able to interact personally and socially. She is requesting a hysterectomy. All other treatment has failed.
Question 26	A 27 year old woman is distressed as she is not able to concentrate in her job due to severe premenstrual syndrome. This is her third job and she is not interested in taking tablets.
Question 27	A 30 year old woman is seeking advice for premenstrual mood swings and bad temper. She is in a new relationship and is seeking contraceptive advice as well.

Answers and explanations

Answer 25 (B) GnRH analogues along with add-back therapy

When treating women with severe premenstrual syndrome, surgery should not be contemplated without the preoperative use of GnRH analogues. This can be used as a test of cure and to ensure that hormone replacement therapy is tolerated. Such therapy should be reserved for extremely severe PMS sufferers in whom other treatment has failed.

Answer 26 (A) Cognitive behavioural therapy

When treating women with severe premenstrual syndrome, cognitive behavioural therapy should be considered routinely as a treatment option.

Answer 27 (E) Continuous contraceptive pill

When treating women with PMS, emerging data suggests that consideration should be given to use of the contraceptive pill continuously rather than cyclically.

(Ref. RCOG, Green-top Guideline no. 48.)

EMQs on Chronic Pelvic Pain and Endometriosis

Options for questions 28 – 29

A	Consider injection of local anaesthetic	F	Refer to psychosexual counsellor
B	STI screening	G	USG scan
C	Refer to physiotherapist	H	Refer to psychiatrist
D	High fibre diet and mebeverine	I	Combined oral contraception
E	Refer to urologist	J	Diagnostic laparoscopy

Instruction: For each question posed below, choose the single most appropriate answer from the A-J list above. The given option may be used once, more than once or not at all.

Question 28	A 19 year old woman has presented to you with cyclical pain of 6 month's duration. She is also complaining of dysmenorrhoea. There are no urinary or bowel symptoms. No abnormality is detected during examination.
Question 29	A 36 year old woman has come to you with a history of recurrent abdominal pain during the last 3 months. She is also complaining of abdominal bloating and a passage of mucus. Pain is relieved by defecation. No abnormality is detected on examination.

Answers and explanations

Answer 28 (I) Combined oral contraception

In women with cyclical pain, combined oral contraception can be offered for three to six months. It suppresses ovulation and helps in relieving pain due to endometriosis, dysmenorrhoea and pelvic venous congestion. Other ovulation suppressing agents such as GnRH agonist can also be given. They can be offered these before diagnostic laparoscopy.

Answer 29 (D) High fibre diet and mebeverine

This woman's symptoms are suggestive of irritable bowel syndrome. She should be offered diet modification and antispasmodics.

Rome II criteria for the diagnosis of irritable bowel syndrome is described below. There should be at least 12 weeks of continuous or recurrent abdominal pain or discomfort associated with at least two of the following:

- pain relieved with defecation
- associated with a change in frequency of stool
- associated with appearance or form of stool.

Symptoms such as abdominal bloating and the passage of mucus are commonly present and are suggestive of irritable bowel syndrome. Extra-intestinal symptoms such as lethargy, backache, urinary frequency and dyspareunia may also occur in association with irritable bowel syndrome.

(Ref. RCOG, Green-top Guideline no. 41.)

Options for questions 30 – 32

A	Complementary therapies	F	Laparoscopic ovarian cystectomy
B	NSAIDs (specifically naproxen)	G	Hysterectomy and bilateral oophorectomy
C	Laparoscopic uterine nerve ablation	H	Ablation of endometriotic lesions plus adhesiolysis
D	GnRH agonist	I	Danazol
E	Hysterectomy	J	Drainage and coagulation

Instruction: For each question posed below, choose the single most appropriate answer from the A-J list above. The given option may be used once, more than once or not at all.

Question 30	A 36 year old nullipara is being investigated for subfertility. She has been complaining of chronic pelvic pain for 2 years. On examination there is adnexal tenderness. A USG scan confirmed right endometrioma of 5 cm x 4 cm x 5 cm in size.
Question 31	Diagnostic laparoscopy of a 32 year old nulliparous woman shows mild to minimal endometriosis. She has been trying to conceive for the last 3 years.
Question 32	A 23 year old P0 suffering from severe dyspareunia for the last 6 months has been sent by her GP. She underwent laparoscopy and moderate endometriosis was diagnosed. Ablation was done but the pain started again after 2 months and although she was started on pills it worsened.

Answers and explanations

Answer 30 (F) Laparoscopic ovarian cystectomy

The woman should be offered laparoscopic ovarian cystectomy as histology will confirm the diagnosis. Removal may improve ovarian function; decreases the risk of infection and may relieve her symptoms. The risks of surgery should be explained. There could be a possible decrease in ovarian function or the loss of an ovary.

Answer 31 (H) Ablation of endometriotic lesions plus adhesiolysis

In women with mild to moderate disease surgical treatment (i.e. ablation of endometriotic lesions plus adhesiolysis) improves fertility.

Answer 32 (D) GnRH agonist

60% of women with dysmenorrhea and 40–50% of women with dyspareunia have endometriosis. GnRH agonists are potent down regulators of pituitary function. After stimulation there is an initial increase in FSH and LH, followed by their depletion. They are believed to function by creating an estrogen deficient state by about 2 weeks after the initiation of therapy.

The rapid induction of an estrogen deficient state as profound as surgical menopause accounts for most of the side effects related to GnRH agonist therapy. Hormonal suppressive treatment, while effective for pain management, has no specific effectiveness on endometriomas or pelvic adhesions.

(Ref. RCOG, Green-top Guideline no. 24.)

EMQs on Pelvic Inflammatory Disease

Options for questions 33 – 36

A	Admit to hospital	F	Coil should be replaced
B	Coil to be removed	G	Laparotomy
C	Antibiotics and manage as outpatient	H	Laparoscopy and drainage of abscess
D	Coil should not be removed in acute cases	I	Total abdominal hysterectomy
E	No treatment is required	J	Salpingo-oophrectomy

Instruction: For each question posed below, choose the single most appropriate answer from the A-J list above. The given option may be used once, more than once or not at all.

Question 33	A 19 year old girl has presented to A&E with a fever, vomiting and pain in the lower abdomen. She is P1 and her last menstrual period was 2 weeks ago. Her temperature is 38.1°C, and there is mild tenderness in the lower abdomen. On vaginal examination, there is cervical motion tenderness and both adnexae are tender. Her pregnancy test is negative.
Question 34	A 38 year old P2 is admitted with a history of pain in her lower abdomen and a temperature for the last two days. You have noticed that she has had a history of chlamydial infection in the past. A transvaginal scan done suggests the presence of bilateral complex masses of 110 mm x 80 mm on the right side and 70 mm x 80 mm x 30 mm on the left side in size. Her white blood count is 20,000/ cmm and her CRP is 102. Her pregnancy test is negative.

| Question 35 | A 28 year old nullipara has presented with pain and tenderness in the lower abdomen. She is afebrile and on vaginal examination there is cervical motion tenderness and both adnexae are tender. Her pregnancy test is negative. She is HIV positive and is not currently on any medication. |
| Question 36 | A 30 year old lady is seen in the clinic as she has had deep dyspareunia and lower abdominal pain for the last 15 days. She is P2 and her last period was 15 days ago. On examination there is adnexal tenderness but no lump is felt. You noticed the thread of a coil during examination. It was inserted 3 months ago. She is requesting removal of the coil. She had penetrative sex 5 days ago. |

Answers and explanations

Answer 33 (A) Admit to the hospital

Women with pelvic infection have a high risk of subsequent morbidity as a result of tubal damage. This leads to chronic pelvic pain in over 40%, infertility in 15–20% and an increased risk of ectopic pregnancy. Pelvic inflammatory disease (PID) is one of the most common causes of morbidity in young women in both the developing and developed world. Around 10–15% of women of reproductive age have at least one episode of PID. In practice, the diagnosis of PID is made clinically. Current recommendations are to start empirical treatment for PID in sexually active women who are complaining of lower abdominal pain and have localised tenderness on vaginal examination.

Ultrasound scanning is useful in identifying a tubo-ovarian abscess, but it is limited in its ability to identify tubal inflammation. The use of power Doppler ultrasound to identify areas of increased blood flow associated with inflammation has shown promise in one small study. The PID Evaluation and Clinical Health (PEACH) study was performed in America with a high proportion of inner city African-American women. The investigators found no difference in reported rates of infertility, chronic pelvic pain or ectopic pregnancy between the two treatment arms and also reported that overall fertility rates in women with treated PID were no worse than those of the background age and ethnicity matched population.

Admission to hospital should be considered in following circumstances:

- surgical emergency cannot be excluded
- clinically severe disease
- tubo-ovarian abscess
- PID in pregnancy
- lack of response to oral therapy
- intolerance to oral therapy.

Answer 34 (H) Laparoscopy and drainage of abscess

Tubo-ovarian abscess (TOA) is a serious sequela of acute PID. As a result of the rising incidence of sexually transmitted disease such as gonorrhea, chlamydia and the widespread use of intrauterine contraceptive devices, the problem of both acute and chronic salpingitis remains a major health concern. Risk factors for TOA are similar to those for PID, such as multiple sexual partners, prior history of PID, no contraceptive use, intrauterine device (IUD) use and low socioeconomic status. Patients with TOA typically present with a history of abdominal or pelvic pain, which may or may not include fever (>38.5°C) and chills. However, a number of studies have shown that a prior history of PID is obtained in only one third to one half of patients presenting with a TOA. The management of TOA changed dramatically after the development of broad spectrum antibiotics. As most women with TOA are in their reproductive years, the usual and accepted approach is conservative; either medical, surgical or a combination of the two, to preserve fertility.

There are three main indications for surgical intervention in patients with suspected TOA:

1. Intra-abdominal rupture.
2. High index of suspicion of other surgical emergencies, such as appendicitis.
3. Failure to respond antibiotic therapy within 48–72 hours. The treatment of choice for an acute pelvic abscess may be a combination of intravenous antibiotics and an early laparoscopic surgical procedure.

Answer 35 (C) Antibiotics and manage as outpatient

Treatment should be the same in women with human immunodeficiency virus. If they fail to respond or clinically there is any suspicion of immunosuppression, advice from the HIV specialist team should be sought. This woman has got symptoms of mild pelvic inflammatory disease and hence can be managed as an outpatient.

Answer 36 (B) Coil to be removed

There is limited evidence regarding removal of the coil in women with suspected pelvic inflammatory disease. The outcome of treatment may be better with its removal. This woman had unprotected intercourse 5 days ago. The risk of pregnancy must be balanced against the benefits of its removal. This should be discussed and as the woman wants it to be removed, it can be.

(Ref. RCOG, Green-top Guideline no. 32.)

EMQs on Heavy Menstrual Bleeding

Options for questions 37 – 39

A	Transvaginal scan for endometrial thickness	G	Progesterone-only contraception
B	Pipelle endometrial sampling	H	Uterine artery embolization
C	Total abdominal hysterectomy	I	Hysteroscopy and biopsy
D	Hydrothermablation	J	Laparoscopic myomectomy
E	NovaSure®	K	Tranexamic acid and mefenamic acid
F	LNG-IUS	L	Combined pills

Instruction: For each question posed below, choose the single most appropriate answer from the A-L list above. The given option may be used once, more than once or not at all.

Question 37	A 32 year old P1 has been referred for heavy menstrual bleeding. Her BMI is 40 and her haemoglobin is 10.5 gm/dl. A transvaginal scan done has suggested a normal sized uterus and ovaries. Her partner had a vasectomy done 3 years ago. The non-hormonal preparation she has had for 4 months has given no relief.
Question 38	A 55 year old nulliparous woman with a BMI of 23 has been referred for heavy menstrual bleeding. She is complaining of intermenstrual bleeding as well. Her haemoglobin is 10 gm/dl. A cervical smear done a year before was normal. A transvaginal scan has suggested a normal sized uterus and ovaries.
Question 39	A 32 year old P3 has been referred for heavy menstrual bleeding. Her BMI is 42 and haemoglobin is 11 gm/dl. A transvaginal scan done has suggested normal sized uterus and ovaries. She is diabetic and was treated for thromboembolism during pregnancy.

Answers and explanations

Answer 37 (F) LNG-IUS

LNG-IUS is the first-line management for heavy menstrual bleeding. Heavy menstrual bleeding can occur for a variety of reasons. It can be ovulatory or anovulatory. Increased fibrinolytic activity, increased prostaglandin levels or the presence of a fibroid can also be causes.

In those with hormonal imbalance (alteration in hypothalamic-pituitary-ovarian-endometrial axis) often no pathology is recognized.

The levonorgestrel-releasing intrauterine system (LNG-IUS) is an intrauterine, long-term progestogen-only method of contraception licensed for 5 years of use. It releases 20 micrograms of levonorgestrel every day. The effects of the LNG-IUS are local and hormonal. It prevents endometrial proliferation and thickens cervical mucus, and suppresses ovulation in a small percentage of cases.

LNG-IUS decreases bleeding in between 71% and 96% of cases. Benefits may not be evident for 6 months.

Answer 38 (B) Pipelle endometrial sampling

A biopsy should be taken to exclude endometrial cancer or atypical hyperplasia. Indications for a biopsy include, for example, persistent intermenstrual bleeding, and in women aged 45 and over, treatment failure or ineffective treatment. Saline infusion sonography should not be used as a first-line diagnostic tool.

A number of biopsy methods are available but the one most often tested in menstrual problems is pipelle curettage. The sensitivity, specificity, PPV and NPV of biopsies for identifying endometrial cancer for pipelle are 70%, 100%, 100% and 99.4% respectively.

Answer 39 (K) Tranexamic acid and mefenamic acid

The risk of using combined oral contraception in women with a BMI 35kg/m² usually outweighs the benefits. Also, the use of combined oral contraception in women who have cardiovascular disease risk factors such as older age, smoking, diabetes, hypertension and obesity, outweigh the benefits.

Non steroidal anti-inflammatory drugs have been used to treat heavy menstrual bleeding and dysmenorrhoea. These agents inhibit enzyme cyclooxygenase and reduce prostaglandin synthesis.

Prostaglandins are implicated in inflammatory response, pain pathways, uterine bleeding and uterine cramps. Prostaglandin levels are found to be increased in women with heavy menstrual bleeding.

NSAIDs should be taken regularly from the onset of bleeding. They should not be used where it is thought that HMB is caused by bleeding disorders. As it is used cyclically, known adverse effects associated with long-term use are reduced.

Tranexamic acid is an antifibrinolytic as it is a competitive inhibitor of plasminogen activation. It inhibits factors associated with blood clotting but has no effect on coagulation within healthy blood vessels. There is no increase in the overall rate of thrombosis within those taking tranexamic acid compared with those not taking the drug. The dosage for menorrhagia is 1g (2 × 500 mg tablets) three to four times daily, from the onset of bleeding for up to 4 days.

(Ref: NICE Guideline, Heavy Menstrual Bleeding CG44.)

EMQs on Contraception

Options for questions 40 – 41

A	1 in 200	H	1 in 10000
B	1 in 300	I	1 in 5000
C	1 in 1000	J	1 in 800
D	1 in 2000	K	1 in 100
E	2 in 200	L	1 in 3000
F	1 in 600	M	1 in 400
G	1 in 900	N	6 in 100

Instruction: For each question posed below, choose the single most appropriate answer from the A-N list above. The given option may be used once, more than once or not at all.

Question 40	A 36 year old P2 has been referred by her GP for sterilisation. After discussion you are going to consent her for sterilisation. She asks you about the lifetime failure rate.
Question 41	A 29 year old P3 has been referred by her GP for sterilisation. She is in a stable relationship and is discussing other methods of contraception. She is enquiring about the failure rate of vasectomy.

Answers and explanations

Answer 40 (A) 1 in 200

Tubal sterilisation is associated with a failure rate of one in 200. Women should be informed that pregnancy can occur several years after the procedure. The most common method used in the UK, the Filshie Clip®, suggests a failure rate after 10 years of two to three per 1000 procedures.

Answer 41 (D) 1 in 2000

The failure rate of vasectomy should be quoted as approximately one in 2000 after clearance has been given. Women should be informed that pregnancy can occur several years after the procedure.

(Ref: RCOG, Evidence-Based Clinical Guideline Number 4, Male and Female Sterilisation.)

Options for questions 42 – 43

A	Danazol 400mg twice daily	G	Increase the ethinylestradiol dose
B	Consider TVS	H	Use 2 POP
C	Mefenamic acid 500mg twice daily	I	Use a desogestrel containing pill
D	Cervical smear	J	Use triphasic pills
E	Speculum examination	K	Endometrial biopsy
F	Reassurance	L	LNG-IUS

Instruction: For each question posed below, choose the single most appropriate answer from the A-L list above. The given option may be used once, more than once or not at all.

Question 42	A 30 year old woman of BMI 40 had a depot medroxy-progesterone acetate injection a month ago. She has been bleeding every week for four days since then. She had a smear done a year ago and it was normal. There is no significant past medical or family history.
Question 43	A 17 year old girl has been referred due to irregular bleeding for the last two months. She was started on combined oral contraception two months ago. She has no significant past medical history. She is requesting a change of pill.

Answers and explanations

Answer 42 (C) Mefenamic acid 500mg twice daily

The CEU (clinical effectiveness unit) recommends that if a woman has unscheduled bleeding on DMPA (progesterone-only injectable contraception), combined oral contraception is the first-line option if there is no contraindication to the use of oestrogen. It can be used for up to 3 months while continuing with DMPA. However, this use is unlicensed. Women who have a contraindication to combined oral contraception can use mefenamic acid 500 mg twice or thrice daily to decrease bleeding. As this woman has a BMI of 40, the use of the combined oral contraception risk outweighs benefits for her.

Answer 43 (F) Reassurance

Bleeding is very common for the first few months when using hormonal contraception. It usually takes some time to settle down and any treatment should be done after three months. Changing to other combined oral contraception is not generally recommended.

Options for questions 44 – 46

A	Take missed pill as soon as possible, continue taking pill, no emergency contraception, no pill-free interval	F	Stop pills, use condom for additional contraception and no emergency contraception
B	Take missed pill as soon as possible, continue pills, use condom for additional contraception and no emergency contraception	G	Take missed pill as soon as possible, continue pills, use additional contraception and no pill-free interval
C	Use emergency contraception as soon as possible	H	Omit pill-free interval and start new pack
D	Take missed pill as soon as possible, continue taking pill, no emergency contraception, take 7 day pill-free interval	I	Take missed pill as soon as possible, continue pills, use additional as well as emergency contraception
E	No indication for emergency contraception	J	Stop this pill, switchover to pill containing more oestrogen

Instruction: For each question posed below, choose the single most appropriate answer from the A-J list above. The given option may be used once, more than once or not at all.

Question 44	A 25 year old woman with a BMI of 28 has come to A&E as she has missed two pills. The pills were on the 18th and 19th days of her cycle. She has been on the combined oral contraception for the last two years.
Question 45	A 25 year old woman has come to the gynaecology ward as she has missed one pill. She has been on combined oral contraception for the last 6 months. She has a regular cycle of 28 days and missed a pill on the 13th day of her cycle.
Question 46	A 16 year old girl has come to the clinic as she is concerned about pelvic pain. She has been on combined oral contraception for the last 3 months. She tells you that she had her period 9 days ago and she has not started her new pack. What would be the most appropriate contraceptive advice to give her?

Answer 44 (H) Take missed pill as soon as possible, continue pills, use additional contraception and no pill-free interval

Answer 45 (D) Take missed pill as soon as possible, continue taking pill and no emergency contraception is needed, take 7 day pill-free interval

Answer 46 (I) Take missed pill as soon as possible, continue pills, use additional as well as emergency contraception

<Below is a rekeyed version of the flow chart found here: http://www. fsrh.org/pdfs/CEUStatementMissedPills.pdf >

Missed Combined Oral Contraceptive Pills (COCs): CEU Advice for Health Professionals

---

If one pill has been missed (more than 24 hours and up to 48 hours late)

Continuing contraceptive cover
- The missed pill should be taken as soon as it is remembered.
- The remaining pills should be continued at the usual time.

Minimising the risk of pregnancy
Emergency contraception (EC) is not usually required but may need to be considered if pills have been missed earlier in the packet or in the last week of the previous packet.

If two or more pills have been missed (more than 48 hours late)

Continuing contraceptive cover
• The most recent missed pill should be taken as soon as possible.
• The remaining pills should be continued at the usual time.
• Condoms should be used or sex avoided until seven consecutive active pills have been taken. This advice may be overcautious in the second and third weeks, but the advice is a backup in the event that further pills are missed.

Minimising the risk of pregnancy

If pills are missed in the first week (Pills 1-7)	If pills are missed in the second week (Pills 8-14)	If pills are missed in the third week (Pills 15-21)
EC should be considered if unprotected sex occurred in the pill-free interval or in the first week of pill-taking.	No indication for EC if the pills in the preceding 7 days have been taken consistently and correctly (assuming the pills thereafter are taken correctly and additional contraceptive precautions are used).	OMIT THE PILL-FREE INTERVAL by finishing the pills in the current pack (or discarding any placebo tablets) and starting a new pack the next day.

(text © Faculty of Sexual and Reproductive Healthcare (FSRH), Clinical Effectiveness Unit, CEU Statement (May 2011) Missed Pill Recommendations,. http://www.fsrh.org/pdfs/ CEUStatementMissedPills.pdf)

EMQs on **Pre and Post Menopausal Cysts**

Options for questions 47 – 49

A	MRI scan	F	CA-125
B	Aspiration of ovarian cysts	G	Laparoscopy
C	Reassurance and follow-up with three monthly scan	H	Reassurance and six monthly follow-up
D	Oral contraceptive pills for three months	I	Reassurance and yearly follow-up
E	Reassurance and no follow-up	J	Urgent laparotomy

Instruction: For each question posed below, choose the single most appropriate answer from the A-J list above. The given option may be used once, more than once or not at all.

Question 47	A 35 year old woman was referred to you by her GP because a transvaginal scan done to look for her coil suggested an ovarian cyst. The scan seemed to indicate that the coil was in place but a simple right ovarian cyst of 43 mm x 42 mm x 36 mm in size was also found. The uterus and left ovary are normal. Clinically, she is asymptomatic and has no significant family history.
Question 48	A 26 year old nullipara woman is seen in the clinic and the scan done has revealed a simple left ovarian cyst of 56 mm x 45 mm x 58 mm in size. Her uterus and left ovary are normal. Clinically, she is asymptomatic and there is no significant family history.
Question 49	A 40 year old woman has been admitted under a surgeon as she has presented with acute pain in the abdomen. Initially, appendicitis was suspected. However, a scan done has suggested a right ovarian cyst with echogenicities of 10 cm x 8 cm x 8 cm in size. Clinically, she is tender on the right iliac fossa and her haemoglobin has dropped from 13 gm/dl to 10 gm/dl.

Answers and explanations

Answer 47 (E) Reassurance and no follow-up

Simple ovarian cysts of less than 50 mm in size are usually functional and resolve spontaneously. Usually no follow-up is required. Expectant management has a good outcome. It is estimated that virtually all premenopausal women, and 1 in 5 women who have been through the menopause, will have one or more ovarian cysts. Symptomatic ovarian cysts are much less common, affecting only 4% of women at some point in their life.

Answer 48 (I) Reassurance and yearly follow-up

A consensus statement was published by the Society of Radiologists in 2010. It suggested that follow-up is not required in asymptomatic simple cysts 30–50 mm in diameter, cysts 50–70 mm require annual follow-up, and cysts more than 70 mm in diameter should be considered for further imaging (MRI) or surgical intervention due to difficulties in examining the entire cyst adequately at the time of ultrasound. A Cochrane Review has concluded that taking the oral contraceptive pill does not hasten the resolution of ovarian cysts and it is therefore not recommended.

Answer 49 (J) Urgent laparotomy

This lady definitely has acute symptoms which could be due to torsion or haemorrhage of ovarian cysts. The cyst is big in size and also there is significant drop in haemoglobin suggesting haemorrhage.

Options for questions 50 – 51

A	Palliative care	H	Radiotherapy
B	Surgical staging	I	Chemotherapy
C	Reassurance and yearly follow-up	J	CA-125 and follow-up every three months
D	Refer to gynaecology oncology service	K	Laparoscopic oophrectomy
E	MRI	L	Laparoscopic cystectomy
F	CT scan	M	Six monthly follow-up
G	Reassurance	N	Laparotomy

Instruction: For each question posed below, choose the single most appropriate answer from the A-N list above. The given option may be used once, more than once or not at all.

Question 50	A 36 year old woman was diagnosed to have a right ovarian cyst of size of 30 mm x 32 mm x 40 mm in size. A transvaginal scan has been repeated after a year, which suggests a cyst of 50 mm x 56 mm x 60 mm in size. It also suggests the existence of an irregular solid tumour with an increased blood flow.
Question 51	A 22 year old woman was diagnosed to have a right complex cystic ovarian mass of 30 mm x 32 mm x 40 mm in size with internal solid component and fat-fluid levels. She is nullipara and has no significant family history.

Answers and explanations

Answer 50 (D) Refer to gynaecology service

The IOTA Group has published the largest study to date investigating the use of ultrasound in differentiating benign and malignant ovarian masses. Using data derived from the IOTA Group, simple ultrasound rules were developed to help classify masses as benign (B-rules) or malignant (M-rules). Using these rules the reported sensitivity was 95%, specificity 91%, positive likelihood ratio of 10.37 and negative likelihood ratio of 0.06.

IOTA (International Ovarian Tumor Analysis) Group ultrasound 'rules' to classify masses as benign (B-rules) or malignant (M-rules) is outlined below.

B-rules	M-rules
Unilocular cysts	Irregular solid tumour
Presence of solid components where the largest solid component >7 mm	Ascites
Presence of acoustic shadowing	At least four papillary structures
Smooth multilocular tumour with largest diameter <100 mm	Irregular multilocular solid tumour with largest diameter ≥100 mm
No blood flow	Very strong blood flow

Women with an ovarian mass with any of the M-rule ultrasound findings should be referred to a gynaecological oncological service.

Answer 51 (L) Laparoscopic cystectomy

Dermoid cysts are bilateral in 10–15% of cases. The composition of an ovarian dermoid cyst is responsible for the variable appearance seen during ultrasound scan. They can range from appearing predominantly solid to predominantly cystic masses. Fat-fluid levels and fat-hair fluid levels are seen quite frequently in dermoids and are considered specific and diagnostic signs. Mature cystic teratomas (dermoid cysts) have been shown to grow over time increasing the risk of pain and ovarian accidents. Surgical management is therefore usually appropriate. Laparoscopy is associated with reduced febrile morbidity, less post-operative pain, lower rates of post-operative complications, earlier discharge from hospital and a lower overall cost.

(Ref. RCOG, Green-top Guideline no. 62.)

Options for questions 52 – 54

A	CA-125	F	Repeat scan in 4 months
B	Repeat CA-125 at 4 monthly intervals	G	Can be managed by general gynaecologist
C	Repeat CA-125 monthly	H	Monthly TVS
D	Calculate RMI	I	Laparoscopy
E	Refer to specialist multidisciplinary team	J	Laparotomy

Instruction: For each question posed below, choose the single most appropriate answer from the A-J list above. The given option may be used once, more than once or not at all.

Question 52	A 52 year old postmenopausal woman has had an ultrasound scan done for suspected cholelithiasis. It revealed a simple left ovarian cyst of 40 mm x 36 mm x 28 mm in size. Her CA-125 is 12 IU/L. She is admitted to the surgical assessment unit and you have been asked to review her.
Question 53	A 60 year old woman was referred by her GP. She has complained of bloating and pelvic pain. An ultrasound scan done confirms an ovarian cyst of 80 mm x 76 mm x 53 mm in size. The cyst is septated and has a solid component within it. Her CA-125 is 70 IU/L.
Question 54	A 42 year old woman has come in with pain in her abdomen. A tender lump of variegated consistency of 24 week size is palpated during examination. An ultrasound scan done confirms an ovarian cyst 12 cm x 9 cm x 10 cm in size with a solid component and septation. Her CA-125 is 25 IU/L. Her white cell count is 17x106 and her C reactive protein is 324.

Answers and explanations

Answer 52 (F) Repeat scan in four months

If the size of the cyst is less than 5 cm, unilocular, without any solid area, the risk of malignancy is less than 1%. Most resolve themselves spontaneously within three to four months so it is reasonable to repeat the scan in four months.

CA-125 is a glycoprotein and is elevated in 80% of cases of advanced epithelial cell ovarian cancer. However, only 50% of patients with a clinically detectable stage I disease have elevated CA-125 levels. CA-125 levels are increased in malignant tumours of the pancreas, breast, lung, colon and ovary. Also, it is raised in benign conditions such as endometriosis, pelvic inflammatory disease and liver disease. The RMI (risk of malignancy index) is an equation used to calculate the risk of a cyst being cancerous.

RMI calculates scores using ultrasound features, menopausal status and preoperative CA-125 level.

RMI score = ultrasound score x menopausal score x CA-125 level in U/ml.

Ultrasound features:

- multilocular cyst
- solid areas
- bilateral lesions
- ascites
- intra-abdominal metastases.

USG score

0= none
1= one abnormality
3= two or more abnormalities

Menopausal score

- Premenopausal -1
- Post menopause -3

Answer 53 (E) Refer to specialist multidisciplinary team

All women with an RMI 1 score of 250 or more should be referred to a specialist multidisciplinary team as there is more likelihood of malignant ovarian cancer.

Answer 54 (J) Laparotomy

This woman's clinical presentations as well as investigations are suggestive of ovarian torsion. Torsion and haemorrhage within the cysts may be seen as solid components and septations.

(Ref. RCOG, *Green-top Guideline no. 34.*)

EMQs on **Prolapse and Urinary Incontinence**

Options for questions 55 – 57

A	Stage 0	I	Stage 1
B	Stage 3. Mainly posterior wall prolapse	J	Stage 3. Mainly cystocele and cervical descent
C	Stage 4. Mainly anterior wall and posterior wall prolapse	K	Stage 3. Mainly anterior wall and posterior wall prolapse
D	Stage 3. Mainly cystocele	L	Stage 2. Only uterine descent
E	Stage 4. Mainly cystocele	M	Stage 2. Mainly cystocele
F	Stage 5. Mainly posterior wall prolapse	N	Stage 2. Mainly cystocele and cervical descent
G	Stage 1. Only uterine descent	O	Stage 5
H	Stage 1. Mainly cystocele	P	Stage 2

Instruction: For each question posed below, choose the single most appropriate answer from the A-P list above. The given option may be used once, more than once or not at all.

Question 55	A 58 year old multiparous Caucasian presents with pelvic heaviness and the sensation of something protruding from the vagina. Symptoms worsen after prolonged physical exertion such as lifting or standing. Increasingly, she is experiencing difficulties in emptying her bladder, and she needs to reduce the bulge with her fingers in order to empty her bladder. She does not have urinary leakage of any type, including leakage during physical exercise. On pelvic examination her POP-Q measurements are Aa+3, Ba+6, C-4, gh 4, pb 1.5, tvl 6, Ap -3, Bp -2.
Question 56	A 60 year old P4 postmenopausal woman is complaining of a lump in her vagina which has been there for the last year. On pelvic examination her POP-Q measurements are Aa+1, Ba+3, C+3, gh 4, pb 3, tvl 8, Ap 0, Bp 0, and D-4. On bimanual examination no masses are found and the uterus is of normal size.
Question 57	A 50 year old Caucasian multiparous woman is referred to a gynaecologist by her GP due to mild utero-vaginal prolapse seen during a routine pelvic examination for a Pap smear. The patient is sexually active and entirely asymptomatic. On pelvic examination her POP-Q measurements are Aa-3, Ba-3, C-6, gh 4.5, pb 1, tvl 8, Ap +2, Bp +5.

Answers and explanations

Answer 55 (D) Stage 3. Mainly cystocele

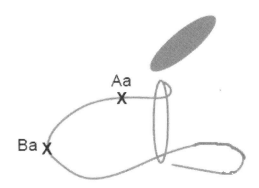

Amended original reprinted from the American Journal of Obstetrics and Gynaecology, 175(1), by Bump, R.C. et al, *'The standardization of terminology of female pelvic organ prolapse and pelvic floor dysfunction'*, pp.10-17, copyright 1996 with permission from Elsevier.

Answer 56 (J) Stage 3. Mainly cystocele and cervical descent

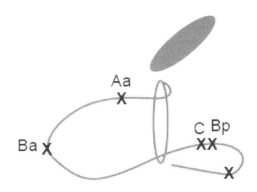

Answer 57 (B) Stage 3. Mainly posterior wall prolapse

	Leading Edge of POP in Relation to Hymen
Stage 0	< -3 cm
Stage 1	< -1 cm
Stage 2	$\leq +1 \geq 1$ cm
Stage 3	$> +1$ cm
Stage 4	$\geq$ total vaginal length -2 cm

International Continence Society (ICS) staging system based on pelvic organ prolapse qualification (POP-Q)

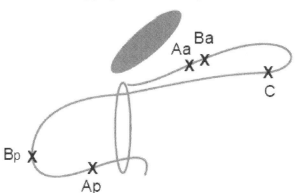

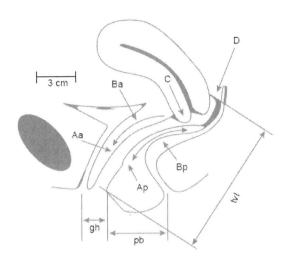

Reprinted from the American Journal of Obstetrics and Gynaecology, 175(1), by Bump, R.C. et al, 'The standardization of terminology of female pelvic organ prolapse and pelvic floor dysfunction', pp.10-17, copyright 1996 with permission from Elsevier.

Prolapses are classified using the international POP-Q system, the process of which is explained by Mouritsen (2005, pp.903-904). "By the POP-Q, the maximal protrusion of two points (Aa and Ba) is measured in the anterior vaginal wall, two points (Ap and Bp) in the posterior wall, and C at the cervix and D at the posterior fornix in the middle compartment [see figure above]. All measurements can be done with a ruler in centimetres. The hymen is used as a reference point (0). Measurements cranial to the hymen are negative, and measurements outside the hymen positive. These six measurements and the length of the perineal body (pb), from hymen to anus, and the genital hiatus (gh) from hymen to the urethral opening are done while the patient is doing a maximum Valsalva [maneuver]. The total vaginal length is measured again without Valsalva.

The nine measurements can be translated into an ordinal stage from 0 to 4 and written in a grid, and for simplification and description of populations translated into an ordinal stage from 0 to 4)."

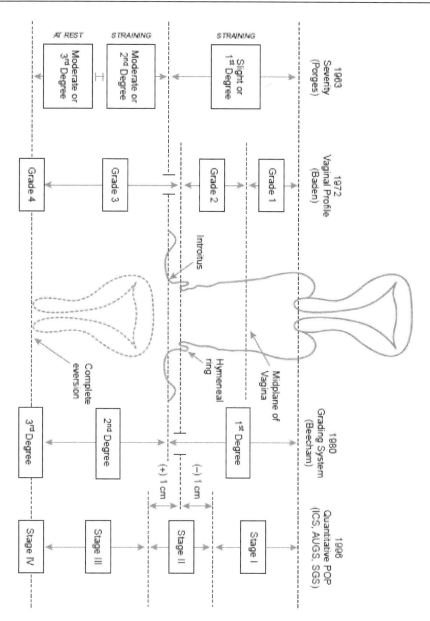

Reprinted from Best Practice & Research in Clinical Obstetrics and Gynaecology, 19(6), by Mouritsen, L. 'Classification and evaluation of prolapse', pp.895-911, copyright 2005 with permission from Elsevier.

Options for questions 58 – 60

A	Solefenacin tablets	F	Urodynamic study
B	Urine culture and sensitivity	G	Sling operation
C	Proprietary oxybutynin	H	Anterior colporrhaphy
D	Sacral nerve stimulation	I	Botulinum toxin injection
E	Indwelling catheterization	J	Tension-free vaginal tape

Instruction: For each question posed below, choose the single most appropriate answer from the A-J list above. The given option may be used once, more than once or not at all.

Question 58	A 34 year old woman has self-referred to the day assessment unit with a continuous dribbling of urine of one day in duration and heaviness and pain in the lower abdomen. She is para 2 and had a forceps delivery 10 days earlier. On examination a lump of approximately 18 weeks in size is palpable. She does not give any history of bowel or urinary problems before delivery.
Question 59	A 45 year old woman with a BMI of 24 has attended the clinic with a history of urine leakage of during coughing and sneezing. She is not able to hold and has had urge incontinence thrice. She is very distressed. She has been doing pelvic floor exercises for the last 4 months without any improvement. Her urine analysis is normal. No abnormality is detected during vaginal examination.
Question 60	A 49 year old woman has attended the clinic with the complaint of increased urinary frequency (14 times during the day and 4 times at night), an inability to hold and she often leaks before she reaches the toilet. Her urine analysis is normal. Her blood sugar is normal. No abnormality is detected during the vaginal examination.

Answers and explanations

Answer 58 (E) Indwelling catheterization

This is a case of overflow incontinence. Bladder atony is common after instrumental delivery. The palpable lump is a distended bladder. Management involves indwelling catheterization.

Answer 59 (F) Urodynamic study

As the patient is having symptoms suggestive of mixed incontinence (both stress and urge), the woman should undergo urodynamic study.

Answer 60 (C) Proprietary oxybutynin

The woman's symptoms are predominantly suggestive of urge incontinence. Urodynamic study is not recommended if the symptoms are clear. She should be offered treatment with antimuscarinics. Proprietary oxybutynin is the first choice.

(Ref. NICE Guideline, *Urinary Incontinence: the Management of Urinary Incontinence in Women, CG0.*)

Options for questions 61 – 62

A	Stress urinary incontinence	F	Vesicovaginal fistula
B	Overactive bladder syndrome	G	Overflow incontinence
C	Mixed urinary incontinence	H	Small bladder capacity
D	Raised abdominal pressure	I	Raised detrusor pressure only
E	No incontinence is demonstrated	J	Raised bladder pressure only

Instruction: For each question (the urodynamic study of two different women who presented with a history of mixed urinary incontinence) posed below, choose the single most appropriate answer from the A-J list above. The given option may be used once, more than once or not at all.

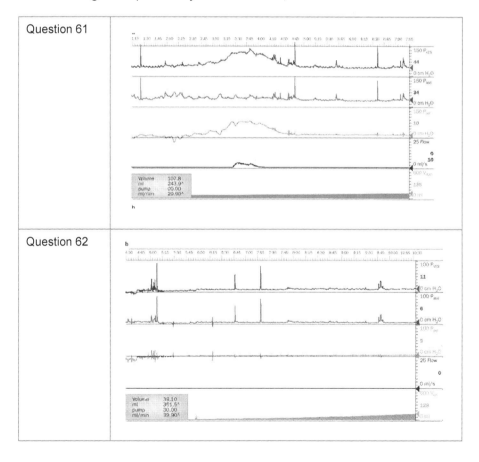

Answer 61 (B) Overactive bladder syndrome

Bladder pressure – top line

Abdominal pressure – second line

Detrusor pressure – third line (subtract abdominal pressure from bladder pressure)

In women who have overactive bladder syndrome there is uninhibited detrusor activity, which is seen as an increase in pressure in the top line whilst abdominal pressure is constant and not increased. Detrusor pressure is increased and is associated with urine flow. Consequentially, the diagnosis is overactive bladder syndrome.

(DO: detrusor over activity; OAB: overactive bladder; P_{abd}: abdominal pressure; P_{det}: detrusor pressure; P_{VES}: vesical (bladder) pressure; V_{H2O}: volume of water; V_{inf}: infused volume.)

Answer 62 (E) No incontinence is demonstrated

In this trace there is no detrusor overactivity and no incontinence is demonstrated.

Options for questions 63 – 66

A	McCall culdoplasty	F	Sacrospinous fixation
B	Anterior repair	G	Posterior repair
C	Pelvic floor exercises	H	Ring pessary
D	Iliococcygeus fixation	I	Abdominal sacrocolpopexy
E	Colpocleisis	J	Vaginal uterosacral ligament suspension

Instruction: For each question posed below, choose the single most appropriate surgery for vault prolapse from the A-J list above. The given option may be used once, more than once or not at all.

Question 63	A 59 year sexually active woman with chronic pelvic pain is referred by her GP. An ultrasound scan has suggested a simple ovarian cyst of 10 cm x 6 cm x 5 cm in size. She had a hysterectomy done five years ago for heavy menstrual bleeding. She is also complaining of something coming down per vaginum. On examination, a vault prolapse has been detected. What would be the most appropriate management?
Question 64	An 86 year old frail woman with vault prolapse is seen in the clinic. She does not wish to retain her vagina. She is hypertensive, diabetic and had a cardiac bypass done a few months ago. What would be the most appropriate management?
Question 65	A 56 year old woman is undergoing vaginal hysterectomy for DUB and uterine prolapse. What should be done to prevent enterocele and vault prolapse?
Question 66	A 59 year old woman is undergoing vaginal hysterectomy, anterior and posterior repair for uterine prolapse, cystocele and rectocele. It was noticed after the hysterectomy that the vault descended to the introitus during closure.

Answers and explanations

Answer 63 (I) Abdominal sacrocolpopexy

Abdominal sacrocolpopexy can be carried out if women require laparotomy for another indication. It has a higher success rate of about 90%. Abdominal sacrocolpopexy is associated with a lower rate of recurrent vault prolapse and dyspareunia than vaginal sacrospinous colpopexy. These benefits must be balanced against a longer operating time and recovery period, increased cost and a longer return to daily activities time.

Abdominal sacral colpopexy uses the interposition of a synthetic mesh or tissue graft between the vagina and sacrum, which allows for more global support of the vagina and distribution of tension over a larger surface area. The procedure has the added advantage over the traditional procedures in that it maintains the normal axis of the vagina, while the maximal vaginal length for optimal sexual function is also preserved. It also provides a source of strength in patients with weak tissue or recurrent prolapsed vault (Uzoma and Farag, 2009).

Answer 64 (E) Colpocleisis

Vaginal vault prolapse is a common complication following vaginal hysterectomy, which has a negative impact on a woman's quality of life. Management should be individualised, taking into consideration the surgeon's experience, patient's age, co-morbidities, previous surgery and sex life.

Colpocleisis is a safe and effective procedure that can be considered for those women who do not wish to retain sexual function. The procedure can also be performed under local anaesthesia, which suits frail women who may be difficult to anaesthetise.

Answer 65 (A) McCall culdoplasty

Various surgical techniques have been advanced in hysterectomy to prevent vault prolapse. McCall culdoplasty at the time of vaginal hysterectomy is a recommended measure to prevent enterocele formation. This involves the suspension of the vault into the origins of the uterosacral ligaments and obliteration of the cul-de-sac. The original description involved an extensive excision of vaginal epithelium, which often resulted in dyspareunia (Uzoma and Farag, 2009). More recently, Elkins et al (1995) described a high McCall culdoplasty.

Answer 66 (F) Sacrospinous fixation

Sacrospinous fixation at the time of vaginal hysterectomy is recommended when the vault descends to the introitus during closure. "The technique comprises dissection into the paravaginal space and the ischial spine is identified... Two non-absorbable sutures are placed through the sacrospinous ligament, one and a half to two fingerbreadths medial to the ischial spine. One end of each suture is attached to the under surface of the posterior vaginal wall at the apical area. When the posterior colporrhaphy reaches the mid-portion of the vagina, the sacrospinous sutures are tied, firmly attaching the vaginal apex to the surface of the coccygeal-sacrospinous ligament complex" (Uzoma and Farag, 2009).

(Ref. RCOP, Green-top Guideline no. 56.)

EMQs on Infertility and Amenorrhoea

Options for questions 67 – 68

A	HbA1c	F	Serum fructosamine
B	Offer a glucose challenge test	G	Fasting blood glucose, annually
C	Fasting insulin and HOMA-IR	H	Offer a glucose tolerance test
D	Fasting and postprandial blood glucose	I	Fasting blood glucose, every six months
E	Fasting insulin	J	Urine examination

Instruction: For each question posed below, choose the single most appropriate answer from the A-J list above. The given option may be used once, more than once or not at all.

Question 67	A 30 year old woman has been diagnosed with polycystic ovarian syndrome. She is anxious about the long-term risk. Her main concern is diabetes.
Question 68	A 30 year old woman has been diagnosed with polycystic ovarian syndrome. She is anxious about the long-term risk. Her BMI is 30 and her mother is diabetic.

Answers and explanations

Answer 67 (G) Fasting blood glucose, annually

Women with polycystic ovary syndrome (PCOS) are insulin resistant, and are at high risk for glucose intolerance and type 2 diabetes mellitus. It can be detected early by offering screening to women with PCOS with an annual measurement of fasting blood glucose.

They are at a higher risk for a number of other serious health conditions including:

- Diabetes, elevated insulin levels, or insulin resistance: About 30% of women with polycystic ovary syndrome will have some problem with processing blood sugar.
- Heart diseases and hypertension: Women with PCOS often have elevated levels of LDL and triglycerides. These factors are known to increase the risk of heart attack or stroke later in life.
- Endometrial cancer: Because of irregular menstrual cycles and lack of ovulation in women with PCOS, there is risk of endometrial hyperplasia and endometrial carcinoma.
- Sleep apnoea.

Answer 68 (H) Offer a glucose tolerance test

Screening of diabetes mellitus in women with PCOS is done by measuring fasting blood glucose level annually. But if blood glucose is 5.6 mmol/l or greater, body mass index is greater than 30 or there is a strong family history of diabetes, then an oral glucose tolerance test should be offered.

Options for questions 69 – 70

A	A free androgen index	F	Serum prolactin
B	Luteinising hormone / follicle-stimulating hormone ratio	G	Serum 17-hydroxyprogesterone
C	Serum T3,T4,TSH	H	Serum cortisol
D	USG	I	Serum 11-hydroxylase
E	Fasting insulin	J	Fasting glucose

Instruction: For each question posed below, choose the single most appropriate investigation from the A-J list above. The given option may be used once, more than once or not at all.

Question 69	A 30 year old woman was investigated by her GP for irregular cycles. Her cycle is of 45 days. A USG shows polycystic ovaries. Her thyroid function and free androgen index are normal.
Question 70	A 26 year old woman is seen in the clinic with a history of irregular cycles for one year. She has also noticed increased hair growth all over her body and acne over the face. Her serum testosterone is 8 nmol/L.

Answers and explanations

Answer 69 (F) Serum prolactin

Diagnostic criteria for PCOS have been the subject of lengthy debates among clinicians. During the 2003 Rotterdam consensus meeting it was agreed that PCOS should be diagnosed if at least two of the following three features are present:

- oligo/amenorrhoea
- clinical or biochemical signs of androgen excess
- PCOS at ultrasound scan.

It should be noted that the diagnosis of PCOS can only be made when other aetiologies have been excluded. The screening tests are:

- thyroid function tests
- a serum prolactin
- a free androgen index.

Answer 70 (G) Serum 17-hydroxyprogesterone

In cases of clinical evidence of hyperandrogenism and total testosterone greater than 5 nmol/l, a 17-hydroxyprogesterone test should be done to exclude androgen-secreting tumours.

Adverse effects are menopausal symptoms, the most common of which are hot flushes and insomnia. Other symptoms are vaginal dryness, mood changes, and headache.

Options for questions 71 – 73

A	Ultrasound guided aspiration of ovarian cyst	F	Ultrasound guided paracentesis
B	Emergency laparotomy	G	Start on hCG luteal support
C	Refer to fertility clinic	H	Manage as an outpatient
D	Refer to foetal medicine clinic	I	Admit to hospital
E	Non-steroidal anti-inflammatory drugs	J	Emergency laparoscopic cystectomy

Instruction: For each question posed below, choose the single most appropriate answer from the A-J list above. The given option may be used once, more than once or not at all.

Question 71	A 30 year old woman has had an oocyte retrieval done 4 days ago. She has self-referred to the gynaecology ward with mild abdominal pain and bloating. Her haemotocrit is 30% and her white blood cell count is 7000/ mm3.
Question 72	A 39 year old woman had in vitro fertilization done 6 days ago. She has come to A&E with abdominal pain and vomiting. Her haemotocrit is 34% and white blood cell count is 9000/ mm3. A transvaginal scan has suggested an ovarian cyst of 10 cm x 8 cm x 8 cm in size.
Question 73	A 36 year old woman has had in vitro fertilization done 4 days ago. She has come to A&E with abdominal pain and vomiting. She is distressed due to abdominal distension and is having difficulty breathing. Her haemotocrit is 43% and white blood cell count is 25000/ mm3. A transvaginal scan has suggested tense ascites.

Answers and explanations

Answer 71 (H) Manage as an outpatient

Answer 72 (I) Admit to hospital

Ovarian size may not correlate with severity of OHSS in cases of assisted reproduction because of the effect of follicular aspiration.

Answer 73 (F) Ultrasound guided paracentesis

Indications for abdominal paracentesis are:

1. Women who have significant discomfort or respiratory embarrassment because of severe abdominal distension.
2. Women who remain oliguric despite adequate fluid replacement, as the relief of intra-abdominal pressure may promote renal perfusion and improve urine output.
3. Women with an intra-abdominal pressure greater than 20 mmHg, as this is suggestive of the need for decompression.

The rate of ascitic fluid drainage should be controlled and under USG guidance (to prevent cardiovascular collapse and to minimise the risk of injury to enlarged vascular ovaries).

Options for questions 74 – 76

A	Testicular biopsy	F	TESE
B	TRUS (transrectal ultrasound)	G	Laparoscopy
C	ICSI	H	Karyotype
D	Stimulation with hCG	I	Transabdominal ultrasound
E	In vitro fertilization	J	Intrauterine insemination

Instruction: For each question posed below, choose the single most appropriate answer from the A-J list above. The given option may be used once, more than once or not at all.

Question 74	A 40 year old Caucasian couple have attended the infertility clinic. A laboratory investigation done by their GP suggests microscopically negative urinalysis of the partner and an ejaculate volume of 0.8 ml with no spermatozoa detected. Seminal fructose was absent. A serum follicle-stimulating hormone concentration was 8.8 mIU/mL (normal range 1–14 mIU/mL).
Question 75	A 31 year old man is seen in the clinic. He has normal phenotypic features with an unremarkable medical history. He has a tall stature (height 193 cm, weight 74kg). Endocrinological testing demonstrated an increase in the FSH and LH levels (26.5 and 16.9 mIU/mL, respectively) and a very low level of testosterone (1.8 ng/mL). Seminal analysis has revealed azoospermia.
Question 76	A 28 year old man has been referred to the hospital with a chief complaint of infertility. He had a normal puberty. Serum levels of testosterone, luteinizing hormone, and follicle-stimulating hormone (FSH) are low. Seminal analysis has revealed azoospermia.

Answer 74 (B) TRUS (transrectal ultrasound)

Absence of fructose in semen analysis suggests obstructive azoospermia. The most common cause of obstructive azoospermia is vasectomy. A congenital absence of the vas deferens is also associated with it. To confirm this, a transrectal ultrasound can be done. Once diagnosed, genetic testing to rule out cystic fibrosis is necessary as it is more commonly associated with it.

Answer 75 (H) Karyotype

Elevated levels of gonadotrophins with low testosterone and azoospermia levels suggest hypergonadotropic hypogonadism. It could be associated with chromosomal abnormalities and hence a karyotype is recommended.

Answer 76 (D) Stimulation with hCG

Injections with human chorionic gonadotropin (hCG) 1500 IU 3 times weekly should be started.

This is a case of hypogonadotropic hypogonadism. The condition is due to the lack of the hypothalamic decapeptide gonadotropin-releasing hormone (GnRH). It is called Kallmann's syndrome when it is associated with midline defects such as anosmia. Diagnosis is confirmed by very low or undetectable serum levels of LH, FSH and testosterone in a prepubertal appearing adult.

Depo-Testosterone is used to treat the development of secondary sexual characteristics and maintain libido. Depo-Testosterone is discontinued for the induction of spermatogenesis. Human chorionic gonadotropin (hCG) 1500 IU 3 times weekly is begun. After 3 to 6 months of hCG therapy, when serum testosterone levels are within the normal range, human menopausal gonadotropin (hMG) 25–75 IU 3 times weekly is added. Sperm usually start to appear in the ejaculate 6–18 months after therapy has been initiated. "Testis size and sperm counts remain lower than normal, but pregnancies occur regularly with sperm densities in the 2–6 million per mL range. Men who fail to respond to gonadotropin replacement may respond to the pulsatile administration of GnRH by pump" (Cornell University, 1997).

Options for questions 77 – 78

A	HyCoSy	F	Transvaginal USG
B	Hysterosalpingogram	G	Outpatient hysteroscopy
C	Endocervical swab for chlamydial screening	H	Hysteroscopy under anaesthesia
D	Hydrothermablation	I	Laparoscopy and hysteroscopy
E	NovaSure®	J	Laparoscopy and dye test

Instruction: For each question posed below, choose the single most appropriate answer from the A-J list above. The given option may be used once, more than once or not at all.

Question 77	A 36 year old woman is being investigated for primary infertility. She has no relevant past surgical or medical history. Her partner is a 39 year old non-smoker with normal semen analysis. Her hormonal profile is FSH-4 IU/L, LH-2 IU/L, TSH 1.7 on D2, and serum progesterone on D21 was 40 ng/dL.
Question 78	A 36 year old woman is being investigated for infertility of a 3 year duration. She has a history of right salpingectomy done 4 years ago. Her husband is a 41 year old non-smoker with normal semen analysis. Her hormonal profile is normal.

Answer 77 (B) Hysterosalpingogram

In this case there was no history of previous co-morbidities such as ectopic pregnancy, endometriosis or pelvic inflammatory disease. According to NICE guidelines, in the absence of any co-morbidity, tubal assessment should be done by hysterosalpingography.

Answer 78 (J) Laparoscopy and dye test

As this woman has a history of salpingectomy, her tubal assessment is to be done by laparoscopy and dye test. In the presence of any previous co-morbidity such as ectopic pregnancy, endometriosis or pelvic inflammatory disease, tubal assessment is to be done by laparoscopy and a dye test.

Options for questions 79 – 80

A	GnRH antagonist	H	ICSI
B	IVF	I	Refer to dietician
C	Clomifene citrate-stimulated intrauterine insemination	J	Gonadotrophin-stimulated intrauterine insemination
D	Metformin	K	Gonadotrophins
E	Laparoscopic ovarian drilling	L	Clomifene citrate and metformin
F	GnRH agonist	M	Intrauterine insemination
G	Advise weight loss	N	Gonadotrophins and hCG

Instruction: For each question posed below, choose the single most appropriate answer from the A-N list above. The given option may be used once, more than once or not at all.

Question 79	A 34 year old woman with a BMI of 23 has been trying to conceive for the last 3 years. Her partner's semen analysis is normal. She has had a scan done which suggested polycystic ovaries. Her serum progesterone on day 21 is 6ng/dL. Her FSH level is 3 IU/L and her LH level is 5 IU/L. She has been on clomifene citrate for the last 6 months. A subsequent scan and hormonal test has confirmed ovulation.
Question 80	A 29 year old woman with a BMI of 32 has been trying to conceive for the last 4 years. Her partner's semen analysis is normal. She had a scan done which suggested polycystic ovaries. Serum progesterone on day 21 is 2 ng/dL. Her FSH level is 3 IU/L and her LH level is 5 IU/L. She has been on clomifene citrate for the last 6 months. She has failed to ovulate.

Answer 79 (C) Clomifene citrate-stimulated intrauterine insemination

Women with ovulation disorders (such as PCO) and who are ovulating with clomifene citrate (World Health Organization Group II) but have not become pregnant after 6 months of treatment should be offered clomifene citrate-stimulated intrauterine insemination.

Answer 80 (L) Clomifene citrate and metformin

Anovulatory women with polycystic ovary syndrome who do not respond to clomifene citrate (with a high BMI of more than 25) should be offered metformin combined with clomifene citrate. This increases ovulation and pregnancy rates.

Options for questions 81 – 83

A	McCune Albright syndrome	F	Constitutional delay
B	Anorexia nervosa	G	Swyer's syndrome
C	Androgen insensitivity syndrome (AIS)	H	Mayer-Rokitansky-Küster Hauser syndrome
D	Imperforate hymen	I	Turner's syndrome
E	Congenital adrenal hyperplasia	J	Polycystic ovarian disease

Instruction: For each question posed below, choose the single most appropriate answer from the A-J list above. The given option may be used once, more than once or not at all.

Question 81	A 17 year old has attended the clinic with primary amenorrhea. On examination she is 159 cm tall and weighs 54 kg. There is no evidence of acanthosis nigricans, acne, hirsutism, goiter, cushingoid features or Turner's stigmata. An examination of the woman's secondary sexual characteristics reveals that the breasts are small and poorly developed with hypo pigmented areola (Tanner's Stage II). Pubic hair is present although the axillary hair is sparse. Examination of the external genitalia revealed that they are of female type and there is no evidence of clitoromegaly. Ultrasonography revealed a rudimentary uterus and bilaterally ill-defined adnexae. At the time of the laparoscopy, streak gonads were seen. The serum FSH is 45 IU/L and karyotype, XY.
Question 82	A 12 year old girl with a negative past medical and family history presented with a 6 hour history of progressive left groin pain. On examination there was a 3 cm mass in the left groin which was tender. She had emergency surgery for a suspected inguinal hernia. The mass was removed. Histology revealed a twisted and infarcted testicle. She is tall with well developed secondary sexual characteristics and on the USG scan there is no uterus and adnexae.

| Question 83 | A 16 year old girl was seen in the clinic with primary amenorrhea. She is 135 cm tall and weighs 45 kg. The physical examination shows undeveloped breasts and a webbed neck. On an ultrasound her ovaries could not be seen and the uterus was hypo plastic. The plasma hormone levels were: luteinizing hormone 29.30 mIU/mL (2.40–12.60 mIU/mL); follicle-stimulating hormone 74.81 mIU/mL (3.50–12.50 mIU/mL); estradiol 15.12 pg/mL (24.50 195.00 pg/mL); thyroid-stimulating hormone 5.92 uIU/mL (0.27–4.20uIU/mL). |

Answers and explanations

Answer 81 (G) Swyer's syndrome

Swyer's syndrome is a distinct type of pure gonadal dysgenesis characterized by a 46 XY karyotype in female phenotypic patients. Patients usually present in adolescence with primary amenorrhoea and a lack of secondary sexual characteristics. The exact incidence of the syndrome is not known and it is an extremely rare condition. The mean age at presentation with primary amenorrhea is 17.6 years. Secondary sexual characters are merely developed. The gonads are usually replaced by fibrous streaks. FSH levels are high with a mean of 80.5.

In Swyer's syndrome there is a mutation either in the YP11 location of SRY (sex determining region of Y chromosome) or in other genes such as SOX9, DAXI, WTI or SF1, which can affect testicular differentiation and also inhibit Anti-Müllerian hormone production.

Answer 82 (C) Androgen insensitivity syndrome (AIS)

AIS, also known as testicular feminization, encompasses a wide range of phenotypes that are caused by numerous different mutations in the androgen receptor gene. It is an X-linked recessive disorder that is classified as complete, partial or mild, based on the phenotypic presentation. The clinical findings include a female type of external genitalia, 46-XY karyotype, an absence of Müllerian structures, a presence of Wolffian structures to various degrees, and normal to high testosterone and gonadotropin levels. Management includes counselling, gonadectomy to prevent primary malignancy in the undescended gonad, and hormone replacement. The karyotyping of family members is advocated because of known familial tendencies.

Answer 83 (I) Turner's syndrome

Turner's syndrome is a genetic disorder that affects about one in every 2000 females born. The symptoms of Turner's syndrome vary a great deal. The most pronounced characteristics of a Turner's patient are her short stature (less than five feet tall) and her failure to mature sexually. Other symptoms may include heart defects, kidney abnormalities, infertility, thyroid dysfunctions, a webbed neck, a low posterior hair line, a broad chest, a small mandible and prominent ears.

Options for questions 84 – 86

A	Oestrogen producing ovarian tumour	G	Autoimmune premature ovarian failure
B	Micro adenoma of pituitary	H	Pregnancy
C	Androgen secreting ovarian tumour	I	Idiopathic premature ovarian failure
D	Turner's syndrome mosaic	J	Hypothalamic tumour
E	Anorexia nervosa	K	Fragile X syndrome
F	Polycystic ovarian disease	L	Post encephalitis

Instruction: For each question posed below, choose the single most appropriate answer from the A-L list above. The given option may be used once, more than once or not at all.

Question 84	A 27 year old teacher, P0 with a BMI of 21 has attended the infertility clinic. She had regular periods until one year ago. Now her cycle is of three to four months and she bleeds for two days. The scan is normal. No positive family history was noted regarding premature menopause, subfertility, smoking, chemotherapy, radiation or autoimmune diseases. Hormonal evaluation showed elevated follicle-stimulating hormone (FSH) (25 IU/mL) and luteinising hormone (LH) (22 IU/mL) levels. Her thyroid-stimulating hormone (TSH), testosterone and prolactin levels were within the normal limits.
Question 85	A 40 year old para 2 (both normal deliveries), has been referred by her GP as she has recently complained of increasing weight gain and hirsutism. She also gave a history of secondary amenorrhoea of 7 years in duration. No other significant medical, surgical or family history was elicited. She was investigated by her GP and her serum FSH was 24 IU/L, which decreased to 14 IU over 4 weeks. Her hormonal profile was repeated again one month later which showed FSH 6 IU/L, LH 6 IU/L, serum oestrogen 380 pmol/L, testosterone 2 ng/L and normal levels of thyroxine, prolactin and SHBG.
Question 86	A 20 year old woman has attended the clinic with amenorrhoea for 5 months. She had her menarche at the age of 14 and her cycles are never regular. She was on the oral contraceptive pill for the last 5 years but she stopped it 5 months ago. She works in a beauty parlour and her BMI is 16.5.

Answers and explanations

Answer 84 (I) Idiopathic premature ovarian failure

In 1% of women, premature ovarian failure develops by 40 years of age (amenorrhea, infertility, sex steroid deficiency, and elevated gonadotropins). Early loss of ovarian function has significant psychosocial sequelae and major health implications. There is a nearly two-fold age-specific increase in the mortality rate of these young women. Pregnancy can occur after the diagnosis of premature ovarian failure as half have ovarian follicles remaining in the ovary that function intermittently (women with normal karyotype). Young women with this disorder have a 5% to 10% chance of spontaneous pregnancy. Thus, premature ovarian failure should not be considered as a premature menopause. Attempts at ovulation induction using various regimens fail to induce ovulation rates greater than those seen in untreated patients. Oocyte donation for women desiring fertility is an option.

Young women with premature ovarian failure need a thorough assessment, sex steroid replacement, and long-term surveillance to monitor therapy. Estrogen-progestin replacement therapy should be instituted as soon as the diagnosis is made. Androgen replacement should also be considered for women with low libido, persistent fatigue, and poor well-being despite them taking adequate estrogen replacement. Women with premature ovarian failure should be followed up for the presence of associated autoimmune endocrine disorders such as hypothyroidism, adrenal insufficiency and diabetes mellitus.

Answer 85 (A) Oestrogen producing ovarian tumour

This woman might have developed idiopathic premature ovarian failure for which she has not been investigated. However, her first FSH was high, which is suggestive of that. When she started to develop an ovarian mass (which could most likely be a granulosa cell tumour or GCT) her FSH level started decreasing. It could be due to the secretion of both oestrogen and inhibin.

GCTs account for approximately 2% of all ovarian tumours and are detected as a pelvic mass in an ultrasound scan. GCTs are hormonally active stromal cell neoplasms that secrete estrogen. Elevations of serum inhibin A and/or B are detected in some patients. Inhibin B is elevated in 89% to 100% of cases. Inhibin selectively suppresses the secretion of pituitary FSH and also has local paracrine actions in the gonads. Patients may present with vaginal bleeding caused by endometrial hyperplasia or uterine cancer as a result of prolonged exposure to tumour-derived estrogen. In addition, GCT is a vascular tumour that may occasionally rupture and result in abdominal pain, hemoperitoneum and hypotension, mimicking an ectopic pregnancy in younger patients. Surgery is required for definitive tissue diagnosis, staging, and tumour debulking. In older women, a total abdominal hysterectomy and bilateral salpingo-oophrectomy are typically performed.

Answer 86 (E) Anorexia nervosa

Anorexia nervosa is an eating disorder in young women. Patients have an intense fear of weight gain, which is suggested by a low BMI for the age.

Options for questions 87 – 89

A	Hysteroscopy and adhesiolysis	F	Laparoscopy and hysteroscopy
B	CT scan	G	Antibiotics
C	Hymenectomy	H	Laparoscopic adhesiolysis
D	Cervical dilatation under anaesthesia	I	Hypophyseal magnetic resonance imaging
E	McIndoe vaginoplasty	J	Ovarian drilling

Instruction: For each question posed below, choose the single most appropriate answer from the A-J list above. The given option may be used once, more than once or not at all.

Question 87	A 32 year old woman has presented to A&E with a history of severe pain in her abdomen for the last two days. She was seen in the gynaecology clinic 3 weeks previously for severe dysmenorrhoea and a scanty period of 4 months in duration. She has had a LLETZ done for CIN3.
Question 88	A 28 year old woman has been referred for secondary amenorrhoea. Her menstrual cycle was normal before pregnancy and her BMI was 22.5. She is P2 and had a normal delivery 2 years ago. However, the placenta was removed manually. She was on a progesterone-only contraceptive pill after delivery, but treatment was stopped after 10 months because of an absence of any menstruation. Since then she has not menstruated. There is no other relevant medical history and no family or drug history.
Question 89	A 32 year old woman has presented 6 weeks after delivery. She had a forceps delivery and a postpartum haemorrhage of about 2 litres. She had a blood transfusion of 3 units. Now she is complaining of a failure to lactate, tiredness and weakness. Blood tests have shown hypothyroidism.

Answers and explanations

Answer 87 (C) Cervical dilatation under anaesthesia

Answer 88 (A) Hysteroscopy and adhesiolysis

This is a case of Asherman's syndrome. Hysteroscopy will diagnose the condition. After adhesiolysis, a coil is inserted to keep the cavity open and reduce the adhesion.

Answer 89 (I) Hypophyseal magnetic resonance imaging

This is a case of postpartum pituitary necrosis (Sheehan's syndrome), which is a rare complication of postpartum haemorrhage. This is caused by an infarction in the adenohypophysis, usually precipitated by massive uterine haemorrhage. Massive or submassive ischaemic necrosis of the adenohypophysis results in acute pituitary failure. The diagnosis can be erratic and is often delayed. A majority of patients have a slowly progressive course with the gradual onset of pituitary hormone deficiency over a period of many years with variable clinical manifestations. It is characterised by agalactia, severe hypoglycemia and low serum levels of thyroid hormones, cortico-adrenal hormones, and gonadotropin (FSH, LH). The hypophyseal magnetic resonance imaging confirms the diagnosis of hypopituitarism secondary to pituitary necrosis. The clinical presentation varies and is dependent on the age of the patient, rapidity of onset, nature and causes of the pathological process, and the proportion of affected pituitary cells. Mild hypopituitarism can remain undetected for years. In such cases pituitary hormone reserves are impaired while their normal basal levels are maintained. A complete loss of adenohypophysis function is life-threatening and requires immediate treatment.

EMQs on Benign and Malignant Disorders

Options for questions 90 – 92

A	Liquid-based cytology	F	CT scan
B	Outpatient hysteroscopy and biopsy	G	Hysteroscopy and biopsy under anaesthesia
C	D&C	H	HyCoSy
D	Transabdominal ultrasound	I	Hysteroscopy and polypectomy
E	MRI	J	Surgical staging

Instruction: For each question posed below, choose the single most appropriate answer from the A-J list above. The given option may be used once, more than once or not at all.

Question 90	A 60 year old woman has attended the clinic with postmenopausal bleeding. She had previously undergone a unilateral mastectomy for breast cancer and has been on tamoxifen for the last 2 years.
Question 91	A 50 year old P2 (IVF conception) woman is seen in the clinic having suffered from heavy bleeding for the last 6 months. Her BMI is 40 and she has had PCOS. It was difficult to do a pipelle procedure in the clinic.
Question 92	A 62 year old is seen in the clinic with postmenopausal bleeding. A USG done suggests an endometrial polyp. She is nullipara and a diabetic on insulin.

Answers and explanations

Answer 90 (B) Outpatient hysteroscopy and biopsy

Patients with breast cancer are at an increased risk of endometrial cancer regardless of endocrine therapy. Tamoxifen use is one of the risk factors for the development of endometrial cancer. The risk rises with increases in dose and duration of tamoxifen use. Ultrasonography cannot differentiate cancer from other tamoxifen-related thickening of the endometrium. Hysteroscopy and biopsy is the first-line investigation in those women who have had postmenopausal bleeding.

Answer 91 (G) Hysteroscopy and biopsy under anaesthesia

The woman has had a history of infertility, PCOS and increased BMI. As an outpatient, using the pipelle is difficult, hysteroscopy and biopsy under anaesthesia should be done. Obesity is now clearly established as an extremely important cause of endometrial cancer, both in pre-menopausal and post-menopausal women. If the obesity is associated with infertility or amenorrhea the risk of endometrial cancer is particularly high.

Risk factors are:

- high levels of estrogen, endometrial hyperplasia
- obesity, hypertension, diabetes
- polycystic ovary syndrome
- nulliparity, infertility, early menarche, late menopause
- tamoxifen, breast cancer
- functional ovarian tumour, unopposed estrogen therapy.

Answer 92 (I) Hysteroscopy and polypectomy

Options for questions 93 – 95

A	MRI	G	CT
B	Repeat TVS	H	Diagnostic hysteroscopy
C	Reassurance	I	Surgical staging
D	Pipelle biopsy	J	Doppler
E	D&C	K	Diagnostic laparoscopy
F	TAH, BSO and removal of vaginal cuff	L	TAH and BSO

Instruction: For each question posed below, choose the single most appropriate answer from the A-L list above. The given option may be used once, more than once or not at all.

Question 93	A 55 year old woman was reviewed in the surgical ward as her scan suggested an endometrial thickness of 9 mm. She was admitted with left iliac fossa pain. Her scan was done to rule out any pelvic pathology. She had the menopause 5 years ago and is completely asymptomatic.
Question 94	An 80 year old lady has attended the gynaecology clinic as she had postmenopausal bleeding 6 weeks ago. A scan arranged by her GP suggests an endometrial thickness of 6 mm.
Question 95	A 46 year old, para three, woman is very anxious when seen in the clinic. She has had heavy bleeding for the last 7 months and in her scan the endometrial thickness is 7 mm. A pipelle biopsy done has suggested atypical endometrial hyperplasia.

Answers and explanations

Answer 93 (D) Pipelle biopsy

Answer 94 (D) Pipelle biopsy

In a postmenopausal woman with vaginal bleeding, the risk of cancer is approximately 7.3% if her endometrium is thick (>5 mm) and <0.07% if her endometrium is thin (< or = 5 mm).

Answer 95 (L) TAH and BSO

Meta-analysis of 7914 women has shown that pipelle biopsies have the highest sensitivity (81%) for overall detection of atypical endometrial hyperplasia. Simple or complex endometrial hyperplasia in the absence of cytological atypia can be treated conservatively as the risk of progression to carcinoma is extremely low. Where fertility or significant surgical risk is not an issue, complex hyperplasia with atypia should be managed by hysterectomy in view of the risk of coexisting malignancy or progression to cancer. Most women with atypical hyperplasia should have a hysterectomy and bilateral salpingo-oophrectomy because of coexistent carcinoma. Also, there is a 25% risk of progression to cancer. Younger women who wish to preserve their fertility may be managed with medical therapy and repeat endometrial sampling.

Options for questions 96 – 97

A	Cervical conisation	H	Hysterectomy
B	Refer to higher centre	I	Hydrothermablation
C	Referred for colposcopy	J	Offer electrocautery
D	Test should be repeated in 6 months	K	Test should be repeated in 2 months
E	Cervical biopsy	L	Offer large loop excision of transformation zone
F	Clinical staging to be done	M	Offer cryocauterization
G	Examination under anaesthesia	N	Test should be repeated immediately

Instruction: For each option posed below, choose the single most appropriate investigation from the A-N list above. The given option may be used once, more than once or not at all.

Question 96	A 30 year old woman has had a cervical smear done by her GP. A borderline nuclear change in the endocervical cells has been reported.
Question 97	A cervical smear of a 45 year old woman has been reported with borderline changes in the endocervical cells. Her previous smear was done 3 years ago and it was normal.

Answer 96 (C) Referred for colposcopy

Women should be referred for colposcopy after one test has reported as borderline a nuclear change in the endocervical cells.

Answer 97 (D) Test should be repeated in 6 months

Women should be referred for colposcopy after three tests reported as borderline a change in squamous cells. After one test the smear should be repeated, preferably within 6 months.

A summary of standards from the NHSCSP's publication Colposcopy and Programme Management: guidelines for the NHS cervical screening programme, published in May 2010, is described below. Most women should be seen within 2 to 8 weeks depending on the severity.

1. Referral should be made for colposcopy after three consecutive inadequate samples. 90% of women should be seen within eight weeks of referral.
2. Colposcopy should be performed after three tests show as borderline nuclear change in squamous cells. 90% of women should be seen within 8 weeks of referral.
3. Women should have a colposcopy after one test reports a borderline nuclear change in endocervical cells. 90% of women should be seen within eight weeks of referral.
4. Colposcopy should be performed if they have had three tests reported as abnormal at any grade in a 10 year period. 90% of women should be seen in eight weeks of referral.
5. Women should have a colposcopy after one mild dyskaryosis (test can be repeated before referral) but must be referred after two tests reported mild dyskaryosis. 90% of women should be seen within eight weeks of referral.
6. Colposcopy should be performed after one test reported moderate dyskaryosis (100%) and seen within four weeks of referral (90%).
7. Women must be referred for colposcopy after one test reported severe dyskaryosis (100%). They should be seen within four weeks of referral (90%).
8. A woman should be referred within 62 days to the cancer pathway with a high grade cytological abnormality. Once cancer has been excluded these women must enter the 18 week pathway (100%).

9.   100% of women must be referred for colposcopy after one test reported as possible invasion and seen in 2 weeks at least in 90% of cases.

10. 100% of women must be referred for colposcopy with possible glandular neoplasia and should be seen urgently within two weeks in 90% of cases.

11. Women should be referred for colposcopy if they have been treated for CIN and have not been returned to routine recall and a subsequent test is reported mild dyskaryosis or worse (100%).

Options for questions 98 – 101

A	Chancroid	F	Lichen sclerosus
B	Chronic dermatitis	G	Acute dermatitis
C	Invasive squamous cell carcinoma	H	Lymphogranuloma venereum
D	VIN 3	I	Lichen planus
E	Paget's disease of the vulva	J	Syphilis

Instruction: For each question posed below, choose the single most appropriate answer from the A-J list above. The given option may be used once, more than once or not at all.

Question 98	A 46 year old has attended the clinic complaining of itching around her vulval region for the last 3 months. On examination there is a marked shrinkage and absorption of the labia minora. The histology shows marked epidermal thinning with a loss of rete ridges and vacuolation of the basal cells.
Question 99	A 34 year old is seen in the specialist vulval clinic with itching. Clinical examinations showed a white patterned area which is elevated and thickened (Wickham striae). Histopathology shows liquefactive degeneration of the basal epidermal layer, long and pointed rete ridges, acanthosis and a dense dermal infiltrate of lymphocyte. On her right lower leg there are papules with an overlying white lacy pattern appearance.
Question 100	A 56 year old was seen in the clinic with the complaint of an eczematoid lesion over the vulva. Histology shows large round atypical cells with oval nuclei and pale cytoplasm singly or within clusters among the basal cells of the epidermis.
Question 101	A 30 year old woman is seen in the clinic with an ulcer on her vulva. The ulcer is painful with a sharp defined border. The base of the ulcer is yellowish grey and bleeds easily. She has recently visited Bangladesh.

Answers and explanations

Answer 98 (F) Lichen sclerosus

This is an autoimmune condition. Around 40% of women with lichen sclerosus have or go on to develop another autoimmune condition. The skin is often atrophic, classically demonstrating subepithelial haemorrhages (ecchymoses), and it may split easily.

Answer 99 (I) Lichen planus

Lichen planus usually affects mucosal lesion. It has polygonal flat-topped violaceous purpuric plaques and papules with a fine white reticular pattern (Wickham striae). In the genital area it is more erosive. The etiology is unknown and it may be autoimmune.

Answer 100 (E) Paget's disease of the vulva

Paget's disease of the vulva is uncommon. The most common presenting complaint is pruritis. The prognosis for primary extra-mammary PD confined to the epidermis (IEP) is excellent. It is most commonly seen in postmenopausal, Caucasian females and appears clinically red, eczematous and pruriginous. It is multicentric in nature. The Paget's cells are larger than keratinocytes, have clear chromatin, a prominent nucleolus and grey-blue cytoplasm and they may appear vacuolated with hematoxylin and eosin staining. Many patients undergo multiple surgical procedures, including wide local excision, simple vulvectomy or radical vulvectomy. However, the margins of primary surgical specimens are positive in more than half of the patients. Consequently, the recurrence rate is about 47%.

Answer 101 (A) Chancroid

The disease is found mainly in developing and third world countries. It is sexually transmitted and is caused by bacteria called haemophilus ducreyi. The most common sites are the labia majora and vagina and a kissing ulcer may develop. About half of the people who are infected with a chancroid will develop enlarged inguinal lymph nodes.

Options for questions 102 – 104

A	IA	F	IVA
B	IIA	G	IIIB
C	IIIC1	H	IB
D	II	I	IIIC2
E	IIB	J	IIIA

Instruction: For each question posed below, choose the single most appropriate answer from the A-J list above. The given option may be used once, more than once or not at all.

Question 102	A 49 year old woman has undergone surgical staging for endometrial cancer. On examination it is found that both the para aortic and pelvic lymph nodes are involved.
Question 103	A 70 year old woman has had a TAH and a BSO done for atypical endometrial hyperplasia. Histology confirms it to be invasive cancer with the involvement of the endocervical glands.
Question 104	A 60 year old woman has undergone surgical staging for endometrial cancer. There was adnexae involvement and it was staged as IIIA. Fluid sent for cytology is positive for malignant cells.

Answers and explanations

Answer 102 (I) IIIC2

Carcinoma of the Endometrium (Staging FIGO 2009)

- IA tumour confined to the uterus, no or < ½ myometrial invasion
- IB tumour confined to the uterus, > ½ myometrial invasion
- II cervical stromal invasion, but not the beyond uterus
- IIIA tumour invades serosa or adnexae
- IIIB vaginal and/or parametrial involvement
- IIIC1 pelvic node involvement
- IIIC2 para-aortic involvement
- IVA tumour invasion bladder and/or bowel mucosa
- IVB distant metastases including abdominal metastases and/or inguinal lymph nodes.

Answer 103 (H) IB

Endocervical glandular involvement only should be considered as stage 1 and no longer stage II.

Answer 104 (J) IIIA

Positive cytology has to be reported separately without changing the stage.

Options for questions 105 – 107

A	Surgical staging	F	Reassurance
B	Follow-up with tumour marker and TVS scan	G	Offer salpingo-oophrectomy once family is complete
C	Bilateral oophrectomy	H	Multidisciplinary meeting
D	Offer TAH and BSO	I	Offer TAH, BSO once family is complete
E	Refer to cancer centre	J	Chemotherapy

Instruction: For each question posed below, choose the single most appropriate answer from the A-J list above. The given option may be used once, more than once or not at all.

Question 105	A 30 year old woman was found to have an ovarian cyst of 4 cm x 3.5 cm x 3.8 cm in size. There were few septations and solid areas. Her CA-125 was 6 IU/L. She underwent left salpingo-oophrectomy and the right ovary was normal. Histopathology confirms it to be a borderline serous tumour.
Question 106	A 36 year old woman was investigated for infertility and the scan done suggested an ovarian cyst with echogenicity of 5 cm x 3 cm x 4.5 cm in size. She underwent oophrectomy but the cyst ruptured during surgery. Histopathology confirms it to be a serous borderline tumour. She conceived one month after surgery and delivered at term.
Question 107	A 52 year old premenopausal woman has undergone cystectomy for an ovarian cyst of 60 mm x 40 mm x 34 mm in size. Her CA-125 is normal. She wanted conservative surgery. Histopathology confirms it to be a papillary serous borderline tumour. She is very anxious and you are going to review her in the clinic.

Answers and explanations

Answer 105 (G) Offer salpingo-oophrectomy once family is complete

About 9–15% of all serous neoplasms are of a borderline type. Because of the highly favourable prognosis for patients with serous borderline tumours, treatment has increasingly become more conservative. Complete surgical staging is of great importance. Treatment with surgery alone with long-term follow-up to detect late recurrences is required. Conservation of fertility is often an issue in view of the relatively young age of many patients. About 15% of patients with Stage IA tumours treated by unilateral salpingo-oophrectomy develop a second primary borderline tumour in the preserved contralateral ovary. The behaviour of ovarian serous borderline tumours and the significance of various prognostic factors are unclear and difficult to evaluate. The absence of obvious stromal invasion is a principal diagnostic criterion for borderline tumours.

Answer 106 (G) Offer salpingo-oophrectomy once family is complete

Answer 107 (D) Offer total abdominal hysterectomy and salpingo-oophrectomy

Options for questions 108 – 110

A	Mucinous cell tumour	F	Brenner cell tumour
B	Germ cell tumour	G	Sertoli-Leydig cell tumour
C	Endometroid tumour	H	Granulosa cell tumour
D	Clear cell tumour	I	Struma ovarii
E	Primary choriocarcinoma	J	Endodermal sinus tumour

Instruction: For each question posed below, choose the single most appropriate answer from the A-J list above. The given option may be used once, more than once or not at all.

Question 108	A 40 year old woman has got severe endometriosis. Her mother died of an ovarian carcinoma. What type of ovarian cancer is most commonly associated with endometriosis?
Question 109	A 15 year old girl is being investigated for primary amenorrhoea. Her uterus and ovaries were not seen in the scan. She is tall with well developed secondary sexual characteristics. Her karyotype is XXY. What type of cancer is she at risk of?
Question 110	A 30 year old nulliparous woman has presented with a lump in her abdomen. On examination there is a solid mass of 20 weeks in size originating from her pelvis. The USG scan confirms it to be ovarian in origin. Her serum alpha-fetoprotein is markedly raised. What is the most likely diagnosis?

Answers and explanations

Answer 108 (D) Clear cell cancer

Clear cell carcinoma of the ovary is composed of glycogen-containing clear cells, hobnail cells, and occasionally other cell types. Clear cell carcinoma exhibits unique clinical features such as a high incidence of stage I disease, a large pelvic mass, association with thromboembolic complications, and hypercalcemia. Clear cell carcinoma is also frequently associated with endometriosis, and atypical endometriosis is considered a premalignant condition.

Answer 109 (B) Germ cell tumour

Germ cell neoplasms arise from primitive germ cells. They constitute the second largest group of ovarian neoplasms (~20%). Dysgerminoma is the most common germ cell tumour. In adults, the vast majority of germ cell tumours are benign. The only known risk factor for extra gonadal germ cell tumours is Klinefelter syndrome (47XXY), which is associated with mediastinal nonseminomatous germ cell tumours.

Classification of germ cell neoplasms is as follows:

teratoma
dysgerminoma
yolk sac tumour (endodermal sinus tumour)
embryonal carcinoma
choriocarcinoma.

Answer 110 (J) Endodermal sinus tumour

Endodermal sinus tumour is the second most common malignant ovarian germ cell tumour. This occurs in childhood, adolescence, and adult life (mostly <30 years) and is almost always a unilateral solid or solid and cystic tumour. The classic pattern shows perivascular formations (Schiller-Duval bodies) and eosinophilic globules that contain AFP. It is associated with elevated serum AFP levels. This is a highly malignant neoplasm that is radio-resistant but responds to combination chemotherapy.

Options for questions 111 – 114

A	Cold knife cone biopsy	F	Radical electro-diathermy
B	Simple hysterectomy	G	LLETZ
C	Radical vaginal trachelectomy	H	Chemoradiation
D	Radical hysterectomy	I	Palliative radiotherapy
E	Simple trachelectomy	J	Chemotherapy

Instruction: For each question posed below, choose the single most appropriate answer from the A-J list above. The given option may be used once, more than once or not at all.

Question 111	A 35 year old nullipara was seen in the clinic with inter-menstrual bleeding and vaginal discharge. A subsequent pap smear suggested severe dyskaryosis. Colposcopy and a biopsy confirms it to be invasive cancer. The clinical stage is IB1 and the tumour is less than 2 cm in size. The woman wants to conserve her fertility.
Question 112	A 40 year old nullipara has undergone radical trachelectomy for invasive cervical cancer. Clinical staging was stage IA2. Histopathological examination showed a tumour of 3 cm in size and deep cervical stromal invasion. What would be the most appropriate management?
Question 113	A 42 year old woman was seen in the colposcopy clinic as her smear had suggested moderate dyskaryosis. Biopsy confirms it to be invasive cancer. Clinical staging suggested it to be IB1. The tumour size is approximately 3 cm.
Question 114	A 26 year old P1 woman was diagnosed to have stage IA1 invasive cervical cancer. She wishes to preserve her fertility. On examination she has been found to have a short infra-vaginal cervix.

Answers and explanations

Answer 111 (C) Radical vaginal trachelectomy

Radical vaginal trachelectomy was first reported by Dargent in 1994. It is a fertility-preserving operation for invasive cancer. It is performed in two steps. Initially, pelvic lymph nodes are assessed laparoscopically and metastasis is excluded. The second step is radical dissection of the cervix along with a vaginal cuff and the paracervical tissue.

Indications for trachelectomy are:

1. The woman wants to conserve fertility.
2. Size of cervical cancer less than 2 cm.
3. Stage IA1 and IA2 cervical cancer with LVSI.
4. Stage IB1 cervical cancer.
5. No evidence of pelvic lymph node metastasis.
6. Presence of cervical cancer at least 1 cm away from the internal cervical os on an MRI.
7. Non-neuroendocrine cervical cancer.

Answer 112 (H) Chemoradiation

The recurrence after radical vaginal trachelectomy is 4%. The prognostic factors after surgery are:

- Major
  - Positive pelvic nodes
  - Parametrial invasion
  - Positive or close (<5 mm) surgical margins

- Minor
  - Presence of lymphovascular space invasion
  - Deep cervical stromal invasion (>1/3)
  - Large tumour size (>4 cm)

In the presence of adverse prognostic factors additional treatment may be required. If the margins of clearance are less than 1 cm then radical hysterectomy is recommended. Chemoradiation is preferred if more than one poor prognostic factor is present.

Answer 113 (D) Radical hysterectomy

Radical hysterectomy is the preferred management in stage IBI of tumours 2–4 cm of size in diameter. Surgical treatment (radical hysterectomy with pelvic lymphadenectomy) has the advantage in younger women by preserving ovarian function. It also avoids the complications of radiotherapy (vaginal stenosis, cystitis, bowel damage).

Answer 114 (E) Simple trachelectomy

In the absence of lymphovascular space invasion, treatment options in stage IA1 are conisation, simple hysterectomy and simple trachelectomy. For a woman who wishes to retain her fertility, cold knife cone biopsy is the preferred technique as the margins are not cauterised which leads to accurate histopathological assessment. However, conisation is difficult if the woman has a short infravaginal cervix. In these cases a simple trachelectomy is done. The cervix is transacted 1 cm below the level of the internal os. The insertion of cervical cerclage is necessary as the chances of premature delivery increase due to the incompetent cervix.

Options for questions 115 – 117

A	Management to be deferred till she delivers	F	Immediate radical trachelectomy
B	Radiotherapy	G	Simple trachelectomy
C	Elective CS with simple hysterectomy after viability	H	Colposcopy and biopsy to be done at scheduled date
D	Elective CS and Wertheim's radical hysterectomy after viability	I	Cancel colposcopy and biopsy
E	Cold knife conisation	J	Immediate chemoradiation

Instruction: For each question posed below, choose the single most appropriate answer from the A-J list above. The given option may be used once, more than once or not at all.

Question 115	A 30 year old was seen in the infertility clinic. Her smear was suggestive of atypical glandular cells and moderate dyskaryosis. She was booked for a colposcopy and guided biopsy. A week before her scheduled appointment she called up and informed them that she was 5 weeks pregnant.
Question 116	A 43 year old primigravida was seen in the antenatal clinic at 14 weeks of gestation. She has recently migrated from Africa. Her first smear was suggestive of severe dyskaryosis. Her colposcopy and cervical biopsy which was done earlier is suggestive of invasive cancer of stage IA1. What would be the most appropriate management?
Question 117	A 30 year old second gravida was admitted with vaginal bleeding at 22 weeks. Speculum examination revealed a cervical growth of 1 cm in size. A cervical biopsy done suggests invasive cancer of stage IB1. She wants to continue with the pregnancy.

Answers and explanations

Answer 115 (H) Colposcopy and biopsy to be done at scheduled date

Any pregnant woman with abnormal cytological test results should be referred for a colposcopy. In addition to identifying any suspected neoplastic lesions, this indicates the most appropriate site for a biopsy. It makes it possible to rule out or confirm the presence of stromal microinvasion or invasion. The colposcopist should be experienced in examining pregnant women as cervical volume increases along with the stromal edema and hyperplasia of the glandular epithelium. There is a greater mucus production and the decidual reaction may impair the examination. Among pregnant women, the sensitivity and specificity of directed biopsies, in relation to the final diagnosis of the lesion, are 83.7% and 95.9%, respectively. There is a small risk of bleeding and other complications such as preterm labour and SROM are not common.

Answer 116 (E) Cold knife conisation

Pregnancy does not alter the natural history of cervical cancer. If cervical cancer is found before 16 weeks of pregnancy, immediate treatment is recommended whatever be the stage.

Answer 117 (D) Elective CS and Wertheim's radical hysterectomy after viability

Options for questions 118 – 120

A	Radiotherapy	F	Palliative management
B	Chemotherapy	G	Neo adjuvant therapy
C	Modified radical vulvectomy with bilateral inguinofemoral lymphadenectomy	H	Modified radical vulvectomy with ipsilateral inguino-femoral lymphadenectomy
D	Modified radical vulvectomy with pelvic lymphadenectomy	I	Wide local excision
E	Modified radical vulvectomy	J	En bloc radical vulvectomy

Instruction: For each question posed below, choose the single most appropriate answer from the A-J list above. The given option may be used once, more than once or not at all.

Question 118	A 60 year old woman was seen in the clinic complaining of a vulval ulcer. She is a diet controlled diabetic and hypertensive on medication. On examination there is a 1 cm lump on the labia majora. The medial margin of the ulcer is 4 cm away from the midline. No inguinal lymph node is palpable.
Question 119	A 76 year old woman has undergone a vulval biopsy for suspected vulval cancer. The lesion is of 1.5 cm in size, located within 1 cm of the midline. A biopsy has revealed a stromal invasion to be more than 1 mm. No lymph node is palpable clinically.
Question 120	A 65 year old woman has been referred as she has recently noticed a vulval lump of size approximately 1 cm in size situated laterally on labia majora. The vulval biopsy done confirms it to be vulval cancer with stromal invasion more than 1 mm.

Answers and explanations

Answer 118 (I) Wide radical local excision

Wide radical local excision with a minimum margin of 1 cm of disease-free tissue should be taken. Lesions less than 2 cm in diameter and confined to the vulva or perineum, with a stromal invasion less than or equal to 1.0 mm (FIGO stage IA) can be managed with wide local excision only. Groin node dissection is not necessary as the risk of lymph node metastases is negligible.

Answer 119 (C) Modified radical vulvectomy with bilateral inguino-femoral lymphadenectomy

Dissection of the groin nodes should be performed when the depth of invasion is greater than 1 mm or the maximum diameter of the tumour is greater than 2 cm. A triple incision surgical technique should be used to decrease morbidity associated with en bloc dissection.

In the early stages of the disease, the incidence of skin bridge recurrence is very low. For the lesion situated within 1 cm of the midline (clitoris, urethra, vagina, perineal body, anus), extensive crossover of the lymphatic channels of the vulva may result in nodal involvement of the contralateral groin in addition to the ipsilateral groin nodes. Therefore, bilateral inguino-femoral lymphadenectomy is recommended in a midline lesion.

Answer 120 (H) Modified radical vulvectomy with ipsilateral inguino-femoral lymphadenectomy

In lateral tumours, only an ipsilateral groin node dissection need initially be performed. If the ipsilateral nodes are subsequently shown to be positive for cancer, the contralateral nodes should also be excised or irradiated, as the nodes are more likely to be positive in this scenario.

EMQs on Operative Procedures

Options for questions 121 – 122

A	1 in 100	F	20 in 100
B	4 in 1000	G	6 in 100
C	7 in 1000	H	14 in 100
D	14 in 1000	I	4 in 100
E	23 in 1000	J	2 in 100

Instruction: For each question posed below, choose the single most appropriate answer from the A-J list above. The given option may be used once, more than once or not at all.

Question 121	A 52 year old woman has had an abdominal hysterectomy for a fibroid uterus. In the recovery her blood pressure started to fall and she developed tachycardia. Her haemoglobin dropped and she was taken back to theatre for suspected intra-abdominal bleeding. Your SHO is asking about the risk of this happening.
Question 122	A 51 year old woman is seen in the clinic due to heavy menstrual bleeding. She had hydrothermal ablation done a year ago and it has failed. She is tearful and wants to have an abdominal hysterectomy. She is enquiring about the risk of overall serious complications during the procedure.

Answers and explanations

Answer 121 (C) 7 in 1000

Answer 122 (I) 4 in 100

(See RCOG's *Abdominal Hysterectomy for Benign Conditions*, Consent Advice 4.)

Options for questions 123 – 125

A	4 in 1000	F	4 in 100
B	2 in every 1000	G	1 in 1000
C	2 in every 10 000	H	5 in every 10 000
D	2 in every 100	I	5 in every 1000
E	5 in every 100	J	9 in every 1000

Instruction: For each question posed below, choose the single most appropriate answer from the A-J list above. The given option may be used once, more than once or not at all.

Question 123	A 55 year old woman is seen in the clinic. She has stage 3 prolapse and has been using a pessary. She now wants a vaginal hysterectomy and you are consenting her for the procedure. What is the risk of a bladder injury?
Question 124	A 65 year old woman is seen in the clinic. She has stage 3 prolapse. She wants a vaginal hysterectomy and you are taking consent from her for the procedure. What is the risk of bowel injury?
Question 125	A 60 year old woman is seen in the clinic. She has stage 2 prolapse and wants a vaginal hysterectomy. You are taking consent from her for the procedure. She is a Jehovah's Witness and she wants to know the risk concerning a blood transfusion.

Answers and explanations

Answer 123 (B) 2 in every 1000

Answer 124 (I) 5 in every 1000

Answer 125 (D) 2 in 100

Options for questions 126 – 128

A	40–45 mmHg	F	35–40 mmHg
B	30–35 mmHg	G	25–30 mmHg
C	20–25 mmHg	H	17–19 mmHg
D	5–10 mmHg	I	15–17 mmHg
E	15–20 mmHg	J	12–15 mmHg

Instruction: For each question posed below, choose the single most appropriate answer from the A-J list above. The given option may be used once, more than once or not at all.

Question 126	A 26 year old is having a diagnostic laparoscopy for chronic pelvic pain. There is no history of previous pelvic or abdominal surgery. You are teaching your junior in theatre. What would be the optimum intra-abdominal pressure to be achieved before you put in the primary trocar?
Question 127	A 30 year old woman is undergoing laparoscopic sterilisation. What would be the intra-abdominal pressure to be achieved before you insert the secondary trocar?
Question 128	A 35 year old woman is undergoing laparoscopic salpingectomy for ectopic pregnancy. You have inserted the trocar. At what distension pressure would you like to operate?

Answers and explanations

Answer 126 (C) 20–25 mmHg

A pressure of 20–25 mmHg should be maintained for insertion of the trocar. This pressure results in increased splinting and decreases the risk of major vessel injury.

Answer 127 (C) 20–25 mmHg

Pressure should be maintained at 20–25 mmHg for the insertion of any trocar.

Answer 128 (J) 12–15 mmHg

Once the trocar has been inserted the pressure should be reduced to 12–15 mmHg. At this pressure, distension is adequate for surgery and ventilation.

Options for questions 129 – 132

A	Cervical preparation is contraindicated	F	Outpatient hysteroscopy is contraindicated
B	Routine cervical dilatation	G	Glycine
C	NSAIDs one hour before the procedure	H	Left to the discretion of the operator
D	Intracervical or paracervical local anaesthetic	I	Normal saline
E	Routine use of opiate analgesia	J	Carbon dioxide

Instruction: For each question posed below, choose the single most appropriate answer from the A-J list above. The given option may be used once, more than once or not at all.

Question 129	A 32 year old woman is being investigated for infertility. She is complaining of inter-menstrual bleeding and menorrhagia for the past 9 months. A transvaginal ultrasound has suggested an endometrial polyp of 5 cm x 6 cm. She is booked for a hysteroscopy and polypectomy. What should be the distending medium?
Question 130	A 67 year old nulliparous woman has self-referred to the gynaecological ward with bleeding per vaginum for the last 2 days. She had the menopause at the age of 50. She was on HRT for few years but she stopped as she developed breast cancer. She had a mastectomy done and was on tamoxifen for 5 years. She stopped tamoxifen 3 years ago. A transvaginal scan suggests an endometrial thickness of 25 mm. She is booked for outpatient hysteroscopy and biopsy. She has not taken any preoperative medication.
Question 131	A 38 year old nulliparous woman is seen in the clinic having had irregular vaginal bleeding for the last two years. Her last up-to-date smear was normal. Her scan has suggested the uterus and ovaries to be of a normal size. She is not in any relationship. You have booked her for a diagnostic outpatient hysteroscopy. What should she take for pain relief?
Question 132	A 39 year old nullipara woman has been investigated for a lost intrauterine device. The transvaginal ultrasound has suggested that the coil is in her uterus. She is booked for an outpatient hysteroscopy for its removal. She has uncontrolled asthma. Your SHO is asking for cervical preparation.

Answers and explanations

Answer 129 (I) Normal saline

Normal saline is the medium used for operative hysteroscopy. It is the conducting medium for procedures using bipolar electrosurgery and it causes distension as well.

Answer 130 (D) Intracervical or paracervical local anaesthetic

The application of local anaesthetic into or around the cervix is associated with a reduction of the pain experienced during an outpatient diagnostic hysteroscopy. However, it is unclear how clinically significant this reduction in pain is. Consideration should be given to the routine administration of intracervical or paracervical local anaesthetic, particularly in postmenopausal women.

Answer 131 (C) NSAIDs one hour before the procedure

Answer 132 (A) Cervical preparation is contraindicated

Prostaglandins are associated with gastrointestinal adverse effects and are contraindicated in severe uncontrolled asthma, chronic adrenal failure, acute porphyria, renal or hepatic impairment and breastfeeding. Four heterogeneous trials assessed the incidence of genital tract bleeding associated with vaginal prostaglandins before outpatient hysteroscopy and found no increased risk with the use of prostaglandins. No reduction in the incidence of lacerations to the cervix with the use of vaginal prostaglandins was demonstrated in the three trials.

EMQs on Hormone Replacement Therapy

Options for questions 133 – 135

A	Reassurance	F	Refer to tertiary care
B	Diet modification	G	Refer to orthopaedician
C	Alternatives such as acupuncture and homeopathy to be offered	H	HRT is not the treatment of choice
D	HRT is contraindicated	I	Refer to HRT clinic
E	Take help of specialist nurse	J	Discuss with consultant

Instruction: For each question posed below, choose the single most appropriate answer from the A-J list above. The given option may be used once, more than once or not at all.

Question 133	A 51 year old woman is seen in the clinic with symptoms of fatigue, night sweats and vaginal dryness. She feels depressed. She is P3 and her LMP was 2 weeks ago. A blood test done by her GP suggests levels of FSH 26 IU/L and LH 20 IU/L. She had breast cancer and a unilateral mastectomy was done 10 years ago. She is requesting HRT.
Question 134	A 59 year old woman is seen in the clinic with symptoms of severe backache and pain in her thigh. She is a smoker and her bone mineral density is -2.5. Her sister had severe osteoporosis. She is P2 with no significant past medical, surgical or family history.
Question 135	A 65 year old P1 woman is referred by her GP with symptoms of fatigue, night sweats and mood swings. She feels depressed and hypertensive (well controlled on medication). A blood test done suggests FSH-141 IU/L, LH 96 IU/L. She has a history of endometrial cancer stage 1. A total abdominal hysterectomy and bilateral hysterectomy was done 7 years ago. She is fit and healthy and is requesting HRT.

Answers and explanations

Answer 133 (D) HRT is contraindicated

The decision to use HRT should take into consideration a woman's age, history, risk factors and personal preferences, and for all women the minimum effective dose should be used for the shortest duration. Continued use of HRT should be regularly re-assessed (e.g. at least annually).

Answer 134 (H) HRT is not the first treatment of choice

HRT is not the first treatment of choice for the long-term prevention of osteoporosis in women over the age of 50 and at an increased risk of fractures. However, HRT remains an option for those who are intolerant of, or do not respond to, other osteoporosis-prevention therapies. In such cases, the individual balance of risks and benefits should be assessed carefully. In younger women who have experienced a premature menopause (due to ovarian failure, surgery or other causes), HRT may be used for the treatment of menopausal symptoms and for the prevention of osteoporosis until the age of 50. After this age, therapy for the prevention of osteoporosis should be reviewed and HRT considered as a second choice.

Answer 135 (D) HRT is contraindicated

The new guidelines by the North American Menopause Society (NAMS) have suggested that HRT is contraindicated in women who have a history of endometrial cancer (NAMS 2010 *Position Statement on Postmenopausal Hormone Use*).

The risks of taking HRT outweigh the benefits in women with the following conditions:

- history of endometrial, breast or ovarian cancer
- history of deep vein thrombosis or pulmonary embolism
- history of myocardial infarction, angina or stroke
- uncontrolled hypertension
- severe hepatic disease
- abnormal vaginal bleeding.

Options for questions 136 – 138

A	HRT should be discontinued	F	Patches are better option
B	HRT should be changed	G	HRT is not recommended
C	Options of alternative medicine should be discussed	H	Testing for thrombophilia should be discussed
D	HRT may be considered	I	Isoflavones
E	Oral HRT may be considered	J	Bisphosphonates

Instruction: For each question posed below, choose the single most appropriate management option from the A-J list above. The given option may be used once, more than once or not at all.

Question 136	A 55 year old woman has been diagnosed with venous thromboembolism. She has been on hormone replacement therapy for the last five years.
Question 137	A 48 year old woman is requesting hormone replacement therapy as she is troubled by vasomotor symptoms. She is known to have type 1 antithrombin deficiency.
Question 138	A 48 year old woman is requesting hormone replacement therapy as she is troubled by vasomotor symptoms. Her father and sister have already died due to pulmonary embolisms.

Answers and explanations

Answer 136 (A) HRT should be discontinued

It is recommended that when a woman who is on HRT develops a VTE, HRT should be discontinued. A randomised double-blind placebo controlled trial of oral HRT (2 mg oestradiol plus 1 mg norethisterone) in women with a previous confirmed VTE found that the incidence of VTE was 10.7% in the HRT group and 2.3% in the placebo group within 262 days of starting therapy. It is recommended that if a woman wants to continue on HRT after a VTE, long-term anticoagulation should be considered.

Answer 137 (G) HRT is not recommended

In women without a personal history of VTE but with an underlying thrombophilic trait (identified through screening), HRT is not recommended in high risk situations such as type 1 antithrombin deficiency.

Answer 138 (H) Testing for thrombophilia should be discussed

Testing for thrombophilia should be discussed with women with a personal or family history of VTE.

EMQs on Statistics

Options for questions 139 – 144

A	McNemar test	H	Simple logistic regression
B	Student's t-test	I	Contingency coefficients
C	Wilcoxon's test	J	Multiple logistic regression
D	Friedman test	K	Pearson correlation
E	Mann-Whitney test	L	Kruskal-Wallis test
F	One-way ANOVA	M	Repeated measures ANOVA
G	CHI Square	N	Fisher's exact test

Instruction: For each question posed below, choose the single most appropriate answer from the A-N list above. The given option may be used once, more than once or not at all.

Question 139	Compare three or more matched groups. Measurement is from the Gaussian population.
Question 140	This test investigates whether the expected values for two groups are the same, assuming the data are normally distributed. The test can be used for paired or unpaired groups.
Question 141	This test is for ordinal or continuous data. It does not require the data to be normally distributed. It can be used for paired or unpaired data.
Question 142	This test is used for binary data in unpaired samples. The 2x2 table is used to compare treatment effects or the frequencies of side effects in two treatment groups.
Question 143	This test is used for binary data in unpaired samples. The 2x2 table is used to compare treatment effects or the frequencies of side effects in two treatment groups. It can be used for paired samples.
Question 144	Compare three or more unmatched groups. Measurement is from the Gaussian population).

Answers and explanations

Answer 139 (M) Repeated measures ANOVA

Repeated measures ANOVA (analysis of variance) for two types of study design investigate either:

1. changes in mean scores over three or more time points, or
2. differences in mean scores under three or more different conditions.

Answer 140 (B) Student's t-test

Student's t-test is one of the most commonly used techniques for testing a hypothesis on the basis of a difference between sample means. Explained in layman's terms, the t-test determines a probability that two populations are the same in respect to the variable tested.

Answer 141 (C) Wilcoxon's test

Statistical tests can be used when the data being analysed is not a normal distribution. Many nonparametric methods do not use the raw data and instead use the rank order of data for analysis. Nonparametric methods can be used with small samples. Commonly used nonparametric methods are mainly:

1. Mann-Whitney U test: this is the nonparametric equivalent of the unpaired t-test applied when there are two independent samples.
2. Wilcoxon matched-pairs signed ranks test: this is equivalent to the paired t-test.

Both of these tests have a power-efficiency of 95.5% when compared to their parametric equivalents (this means that the equivalent parametric test would be just as effective with a sample size that is 4.5% smaller than that used in the nonparametric tests). The power-efficiency illustrates the fact that if all conditions of normality (of the sample distribution) are met, then nonparametric methods waste data.

Answer 142 (N) Fisher's exact test

This is a statistical significance test used in the analysis of contingency tables. In practice it is used when sample sizes are small but it is valid for all sample sizes. A chi-square test can be used in large samples.

Answer 143 (A) McNemar test

McNemar's test assesses the significance of the difference between two correlated proportions. Where there are two proportions in the same sample, this test can be used on the subjects or on matched-pair samples.

Answer 144 (F) One-way ANOVA

The one-way ANOVA test is used with one categorical independent variable and one continuous variable. The independent variable can consist of any number of groups.

EMQs on **Medical Ethics**

Options for questions 145 – 148

A	Confidentiality	F	Beneficence
B	Nonmaleficence	G	Bolam
C	Competence	H	Autonomy
D	Battery	I	Veracity
E	Paternalism	J	Gillick competence

Instruction: For each question posed below, choose the single most appropriate answer from the A-J list above. The given option may be used once, more than once or not at all.

Question 145	A 44 year old woman has irregular spotting and has undergone hysteroscopy and endometrial biopsy. Her sister has visited you and requested not to disclose the result if it is suggestive of malignancy. Her mother had endometrial cancer and died within a year of diagnosis and the whole family had a difficult time.
Question 146	A 22 year old G2 who has previously had a LSCS is diagnosed to have placenta praevia. A further scan and MRI confirmed it to be placenta accreta. She is planned for an elective LSCS. She is a Jehovah's Witness and is refusing a blood transfusion.
Question 147	The mother of a 16 year old girl has visited her GP and accused him of prescribing contraception to her daughter. She wants to know when her daughter started taking the medication.
Question 148	A senior registrar was called to review the CTG of a primigravida who was in labour for 22 hours. The trace was pathological and he did a forceps delivery. The baby was subsequently found to have severe brain damage. The registrar was not found to be negligent of duty.

Answers and explanations

Answer 145 (I) Veracity

Principle of veracity (ethics of telling the truth)

A patient must be provided with the complete truth about their medical condition. This includes diagnosis, investigations and progression of condition. This is the only way that a patient can make an informed decision about accepting or rejecting recommended medical management.

Answer 146 (H) Autonomy

Autonomy is defined as the capacity to make one's own decisions. Respect for patient autonomy requires that those with the capacity be permitted to accept or refuse treatment. Patients must be aware of expected benefits, alternatives, and the potential risks and consequences of refusing treatment altogether. The decision must be voluntary and not made under pressure of any kind.

Answer 147 (A) Confidentiality

Essentially, medical confidentiality is respecting other people's secrets (information they do not wish to have further disclosed).

Answer 148 (G) Bolam

The Bolam principle indicates that a doctor or nurse or other health professional is not negligent if he or she acts in accordance with a practice accepted at the time as proper by a responsible body of medical opinion, even though some other practitioners adopt a different practice.

Options for questions 149 – 151

A	Confidentiality	F	Beneficence
B	Nonmaleficence	G	Bolam
C	Competence	H	Autonomy
D	Battery	I	Veracity
E	Paternalism	J	Gillick competency

Instruction: For each question posed below, choose the single most appropriate answer from the A-J list above. The given option may be used once, more than once or not at all.

Question 149	A 44 year old woman is seen in the clinic for an ovarian cyst of 6 cm x 4 cm x 5 cm in size. Her mother died of ovarian cancer. You decide that she should undergo a total abdominal hysterectomy and a bilateral salpingo-oophrectomy.
Question 150	A 15 year old girl has visited her GP. She is in a relationship and is asking for contraception. She understands the risks and advantages of it. She has visited her GP without parental consent.
Question 151	A 30 year old woman was found collapsed at home. She was brought to the emergency department and was subsequently found to have a ruptured ectopic pregnancy. She was taken to the theatre and a salpingectomy was done.

Answer 149 (E) Paternalism

An action initiated by a human individual or group with regard to another human individual or group, is paternalistic if and only if:

1. the action is primarily intended by the initiator to benefit the recipient, and
2. the recipient's consent or dissent is not a relevant consideration for the initiator.

Answer 150 (J) Gillick competency

Gillick competency and Fraser guidelines refer to a legal case which looked specifically at whether doctors should be able to give contraceptive advice or treatment to under 16 year olds without parental consent. The Fraser guidelines refer to the guidelines set out by Lord Fraser in his judgment of the Gillick case in the House of Lords (1985), which apply specifically to contraceptive advice:

"...a doctor could proceed to give advice and treatment provided he is satisfied in the following criteria:

1. that the girl (although under the age of 16 years of age) will understand his advice;
2. that he cannot persuade her to inform her parents or to allow him to inform the parents that she is seeking contraceptive advice;
3. that she is very likely to continue having sexual intercourse with or without contraceptive treatment;
4. that unless she receives contraceptive advice or treatment her physical or mental health or both are likely to suffer;
5. that her best interests require him to give her contraceptive advice, treatment or both without the parental consent."

Answer 151 (F) Beneficence

Principle of beneficence

A practitioner should act in the best interest of the patient.

References

Cornell University (1997) What's new in male infertility treatment at Cornell, http://www.maleinfertility.org/new-treatment.html.

Elkins, TE et al (1995) Initial report of anatomic and clinical comparison of the sacrospinous ligament fixation to the high McCall culdosplasty for vaginal cuff fixation at hysterectomy for uterine prolapse. Journal of Pelvic Surgery, 1 pp.12-17.

Mouritsen, L (2005) Classification and evaluation of prolapse, Best Practice & Research Clinical Obstetrics and Gynaecology,19(6) pp.895-911.

Uzoma, A and Farag, KA (2009) Vaginal Vault Prolapse, Obstetrics and Gynecology International, http://www.hindawi.com/journals/ogi/2009/275621/